# CONTENTS

## ASSESS YOUR BRAIN & MIND

| | |
|---|---|
| **Day 1:** Know the 12 Principles of Amen Clinics | 2 |
| **Day 2:** Use the Science of Change to Your Advantage | 8 |
| **Day 3:** Know Your Brain Type: Brain Health Assessment | 14 |
| **Day 4:** Know Your BRIGHT MINDS Risk Factors | 15 |
| **Day 5:** Know Your Important Numbers | 18 |
| **Day 6:** Know Your Dragons | 22 |
| **Day 7:** Know Your ANTs | 27 |
| **Day 8:** Know Your ONE PAGE MIRACLE and Motivation to Be Well | 32 |
| **Day 9:** 6 Feeling Better Fast Techniques | 36 |
| **Day 10:** Supplement Your Brain | 41 |
| **Day 11:** Brain Healthy Eating | 42 |

## BRIGHT MINDS STRATEGIES

| | |
|---|---|
| **Day 12:** BRIGHT MINDS Strategy: Boost Blood Flow | 52 |
| **Day 13:** BRIGHT MINDS Strategy: Keep Your Brain Young | 56 |
| **Day 14:** BRIGHT MINDS Strategy: Quell Inflammation and Improve Gut Health | 59 |
| **Day 15:** BRIGHT MINDS Strategy: Know Your Genetics | 63 |
| **Day 16:** BRIGHT MINDS Strategy: Protect Your Brain | 65 |
| **Day 17:** BRIGHT MINDS Strategy: Detoxify Your Brain and Body | 68 |
| **Day 18:** BRIGHT MINDS Strategy: Stabilize Your Moods–Mind-Storms | 72 |
| **Day 19:** BRIGHT MINDS Strategy: Boost Immunity to Protect Against Infections | 74 |
| **Day 20:** BRIGHT MINDS Strategy: Optimize Your Neurohormones | 78 |
| **Day 21:** BRIGHT MINDS Strategy: Achieve Healthy Weight and Blood Sugar To Prevent Diabesity | 81 |
| **Day 22:** BRIGHT MINDS Strategy: Sleep | 85 |

## TAME YOUR DRAGONS

| | |
|---|---|
| **Day 23:** Finding Significance: Taming the Abandoned, Invisible or Insignificant Dragons | 90 |
| **Day 24:** Stop Comparing: Taming the Inferior or Flawed Dragons | 92 |
| **Day 25:** Finding Peace: Taming the Anxious Dragons | 94 |
| **Day 26:** Get the Past Out of the Present: Taming the Wounded Dragons | 96 |
| **Day 27:** Does it Fit My Goals?: Do I Want To?: Taming the Should and Shaming Dragons | 98 |
| **Day 28:** Change Starts With Me: Taming the Responsible Dragons | 101 |
| **Day 29:** It's Not All About You: Taming the Special, Spoiled, or Entitled Dragons | 103 |
| **Day 30:** Soothing Rage: Taming the Angry Dragons | 105 |
| **Day 31:** Behavior is More Complicated Than You Think: Taming the Judgmental Dragons | 107 |
| **Day 32:** If It is Meaningful I Do It: Taming the Death Dragons | 109 |
| **Day 33:** Finding Joy Again: Taming the Grief and Loss Dragons | 112 |
| **Day 34:** Finding Hope: Taming Hopeless and Helpless Dragons | 114 |
| **Day 35:** It's Not All About Me, But About Generations of Me: Taming the Ancestral Dragons | 116 |

## DEVELOP RELENTLESS COURAGE

| | |
|---|---|
| **Day 36:** Master ANT Killing: Challenge Your 100 Worst Thoughts | 122 |
| **Day 37:** Write Your Story to Tame Trauma | 124 |
| **Day 38:** Overcome Trauma by Finding Your Purpose | 129 |
| **Day 39:** It's Easy to Call People Bad, It's Harder to Ask Why | 131 |
| **Day 40:** REACH for Forgiveness | 132 |
| **Day 41:** Finding Your Voice: Learning to Be Assertive | 135 |
| **Day 42:** Take Responsibility for Your Life | 137 |

# Week 1

## ASSESS YOUR BRAIN & MIND

To overcome anxiety, depression, trauma, and grief, you need to know more about the health of your brain, body, and mind.

For the next 11 days, we will show you how to discover your brain type, your BRIGHT MINDS risk factors, your Dragons from the Past, and more. With these valuable insights, you'll see that you have an opportunity to enhance your brain health, prevent or treat your risk factors, and tame your dragons so you can transform your life.

# DAY 1. KNOW THE 12 PRINCIPLES OF AMEN CLINICS

**1. Your brain is involved in everything you do and everything you are.**

The moment-by-moment and day-to-day functioning of your brain is involved in how you think, how you feel, how you act, and how you interact with others. Your brain is the organ behind your intelligence, character, personality, and decision-making.

**2. When your brain works right, you work right; when your brain is troubled you are much more likely to have trouble in your life.**

People with healthy brains are happier, healthier, more successful, and better able to get along with others. People with unhealthy brains are sadder, sicker, less successful, and have more conflict in their relationships.

**3. Your brain is the most complicated organ in the universe.**

It is estimated that your brain has 100 billion cells, with each one connected to other cells by up to 10,000 individual connections. It has been estimated that you have more connections in your brain than there are stars in the universe. Even though your brain is only about 2% of your body's weight (about 3 pounds), it uses 20%-30% of the calories you consume and 20% of your body's blood flow.

**4. Your brain is the consistency of soft butter and is housed in a really hard skull with multiple sharp boney ridges, making it easily injured.**

Think of something that falls in between Jell-O and egg whites on the softness spectrum—that's your brain. Now imagine it encased in a really hard skull with many sharp bony ridges. Jarring motions and head injuries can cause the brain to slam into the hard interior of the skull, causing brain injuries that can ruin lives. Traumatic brain injuries (TBI) are a major cause of psychiatric illness and few people know this, because most psychiatrists never look at the brain. TBI has been linked to homelessness, drug and alcohol abuse, anxiety, panic attacks, depression, ADD/ADHD, learning problems, school failure, murder, suicide, domestic violence, job failure, and incarceration.

**5. Many things hurt the brain. Avoid them.**

Based on our brain imaging work and more than 30 years of clinical practice, we have identified the 11 major risk factors that harm the brain and steal your mind. We developed the mnemonic BRIGHT MINDS to help you remember the 11 major risk factors. You'll learn more about them throughout this 6-week course. Here's a quick look at how they can hurt the brain.

- **B is for blood flow.** Blood flow brings oxygen and other nutrients to your brain and carries away waste. Low blood flow seen on brain SPECT imaging is associated with many psychiatric symptoms and is the #1 brain imaging predictor of Alzheimer's disease.

- **R is for retirement and aging.** When you stop learning your brain starts dying.

- **I is for inflammation.** Inflammation acts like a constant fire that harms your organs and can destroy your brain.

- **G is for genetics.** Brain health issues clearly run in families, but genes are not a death sentence. They should be a wake-up call.

- **H is for head trauma.** Traumatic injuries to the head are one of the major risk factors for psychiatric illnesses, even though few people know it.

- **T is for toxins.** Exposure to environmental toxins has been linked to the increased risk of mental illness symptoms, memory problems, and dementia.

- **M is for mind-storms.** Your brain is the world's most powerful hybrid electrochemical engine. It uses electricity and neurotransmitters to help you think, feel, and act. Some diseases of the brain start by damaging the brain's wiring or impairing the ability to create the right amount of electricity.

- **I is for immune system problems and infections.** When your immunity isn't strong, you may be more vulnerable to infections, which can raise your risk of brain fog, mental health problems, and memory issues.

- **N is for neurohormone issues.** When your hormones are out of balance, you may be more prone to anxiety, depression, Alzheimer's disease, and other issues.

- **D is for diabesity.** The word "diabesity" combines diabetes and obesity, both of which decrease the size and function of your brain. Obesity is also associated with greater risk of depression, bipolar disorder, addictions, dementia, and more.

- **S is for sleep.** Your brain needs sleep to stay healthy. Sleeping less than 7 hours a night has been associated with a higher risk of anxiety, depression, dementia, ADD/ADHD, and more.

**6. Many things help the brain. Engage in regular brain healthy habits.**

The exciting news is that many things are also good for your brain and can boost its function. In this 6-week course, you'll learn several BRIGHT MINDS strategies you can use to minimize your risk factors.

- **B is for blood flow.** We'll give you the #1 way to support healthy blood flow for brain optimization.

- **R is for retirement and aging.** You'll discover the best ways to exercise your brain to prevent premature aging.

- **I is for inflammation.** You'll learn how to check your inflammation levels and the best foods to eat to fight inflammation.

- **G is for genetics.** Know your genetic risks. We'll show you how to discover more about your family history and how to use it to your advantage.

- **H is for head trauma.** You'll learn how to protect your head from injury and what to do if you've had a head trauma.

- **T is for toxins.** We'll give you the tools you need to limit or eliminate the toxins that contribute to depression, brain fog, and more.

- **M is for mind-storms.** You'll find out how to avoid anything that increases the risk of mind-storms.

- **I is for immune system problems and infections.** Discover how to strengthen your immune system and fight the infections that can cause psychiatric symptoms.

- **N is for neurohormone issues.** Get simple tips to keep your neurohormones healthy so you can have more stable moods, less anxiety, and sharper focus.

- **D is for diabesity.** Discover how minor tweaks to your mindset can help you achieve and maintain a healthy weight and mind.

- **S is for sleep.** With the strategies in this course, you'll get more restful, restorative sleep so you wake up feeling happier, less stressed, and more resilient.

**7. Certain systems in the brain tend to do specific things; and problems in these systems tend to cause symptoms that can benefit from targeted treatments.**

Knowing about your brain can help you understand yourself and others. There are 5 major brain systems involved with feelings, thinking, and behavior, including: the limbic or emotional brain (mood and bonding), basal ganglia (motivation, pleasure, and anxiety), prefrontal cortex (the brain's CEO – focus, forethought, and judgment), anterior cingulate gyrus (detects errors and helps shift attention), and the temporal lobes (memory, learning, and mood stability).

**YOUR BRAIN: A BRIEF PRIMER**

**Outside View of the Brain**

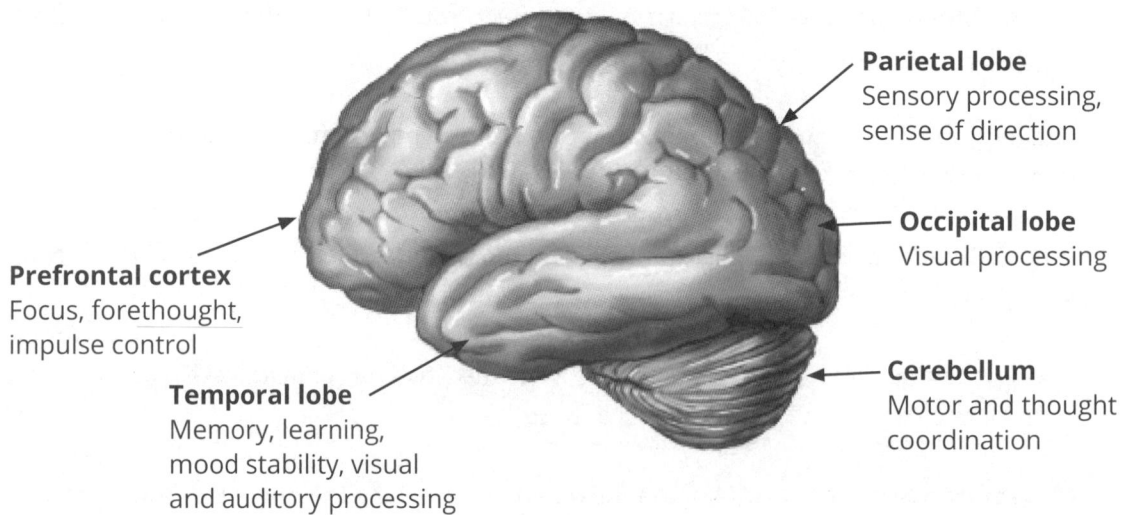

**Prefrontal cortex** Focus, forethought, impulse control

**Temporal lobe** Memory, learning, mood stability, visual and auditory processing

**Parietal lobe** Sensory processing, sense of direction

**Occipital lobe** Visual processing

**Cerebellum** Motor and thought coordination

**Inside View of the Brain**

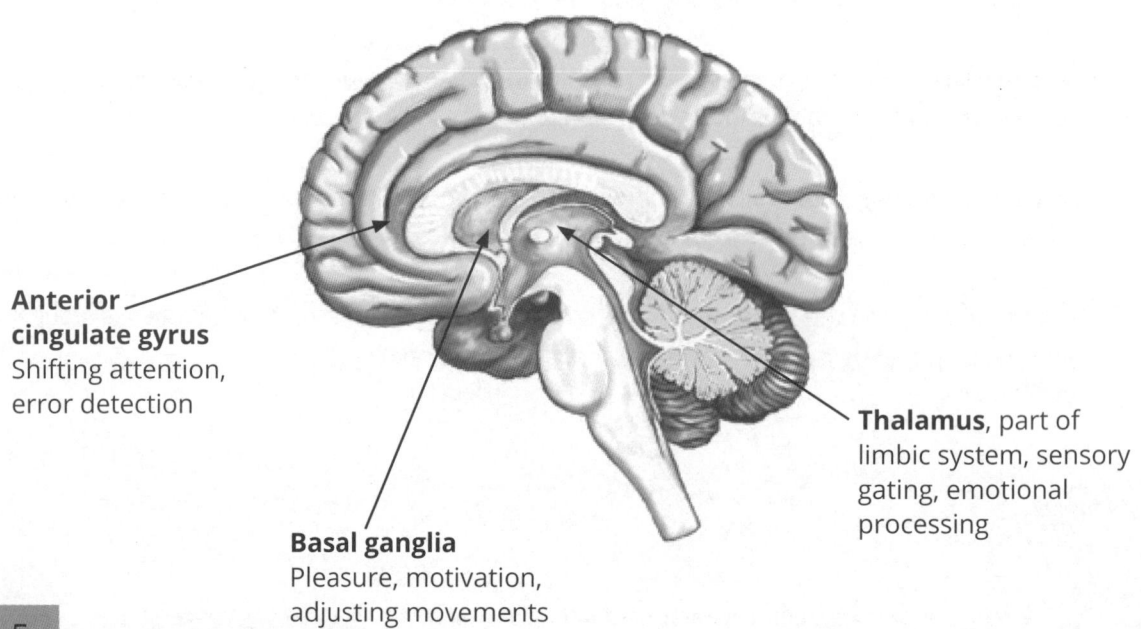

**Anterior cingulate gyrus** Shifting attention, error detection

**Basal ganglia** Pleasure, motivation, adjusting movements

**Thalamus**, part of limbic system, sensory gating, emotional processing

### 8. Imaging changes everything.

Brain imaging helps us stop calling psychiatric problems "mental illnesses," but rather brain health issues that steal your mind. This one idea changes everything. Get your brain right and your mind will follow, which is the big idea underlying this course.

### 9. All psychiatric illnesses are not single or simple disorders. They all have multiple types.

Our imaging studies have shown that mental health/brain health conditions are not single or simple disorders, so giving everybody the same treatment will never work. To discover your brain type or the brain types of loved ones or clients, take our free 5-minute Brain Health Assessment at brainhealthassessment.com.

### 10. The brain gets sick, or gets well, in 4 Circles.

To end mental illness, you need to understand all the factors in your life that can contribute to mental health/brain health problems and optimize them. We call these factors the 4 Circles of a whole life. They include:

**Biological:** how your physical body and brain function

**Psychological:** developmental issues and how you think

**Social:** social support, your current life situation, and societal influence

**Spiritual:** your connection to God, the planet, past and future generations, and your deepest sense of meaning and purpose

### 11. First, do no harm.

We use the least toxic, most effective natural treatments first in a functional medicine context. This means treatments that are targeted for your individual needs. In addition, don't start taking something that you may have a hard time stopping. For example, withdrawing from many anti-anxiety or antidepressant medications can be very hard. Nutraceuticals or medications should never be the first and only thing you do.

### 12. You're not stuck with the brain you have. You can make it better.

This is the most exciting and hopeful lesson we have learned from over 170,000 brain scans. When you take ownership for the health of your brain and mind and put in the work that is presented in this 6-week course, you can have a better brain, a brighter mind, and a better life.

***Day 1 Exercise:*** *Answer the following questions to help put these principles into practice in your own life.*

List 3 ways your brain affects your life.

1. _____
2. _____
3. _____

Why should you care about brain health?

_____
_____

What are your most concerning symptoms you wish to work on during this course?

_____
_____

If your brain worked the way you wanted it to, how might your life be different?

_____
_____

# DAY 2. USE THE SCIENCE OF CHANGE TO YOUR ADVANTAGE

As you begin your journey, we hope you're feeling upbeat and empowered to improve your overall brain health, feel happier and less stressed, and live the life you want. At the same time, we know that lifestyle changes can often feel daunting at first. On this day, we'll share some very simple, science-backed strategies that will help you make the changes you need to achieve the transformation you want.

**1. Know what you want to change.**

Your brain makes happen what it sees. What changes would you like to make? Write them out.

***Day 2 Exercise: Create a vivid and believable "Future of Success" in detail. How will you feel if you consistently engage in the new behavior in 1, 5, and 10 years? You could write: "I'll feel amazing, healthy, energetic, cognitively better than I have ever been, in control."***

Here's an example of how Tana did this:

### FUTURE OF SUCCESS

| CHANGES I WANT TO MAKE | HOW WILL I FEEL IN THE FUTURE? |
|---|---|
| Overcome past trauma | I'll feel happier, calmer, and more in control of my own life. |

| CHANGES I WANT TO MAKE | HOW WILL I FEEL IN THE FUTURE? |
|---|---|
|  |  |
|  |  |
|  |  |

**2. Make a commitment to loving your brain.**

Research has shown that making a resolution or goal and then putting it down on paper (or even better, sharing it with a friend) can help you be more successful, especially when your initial enthusiasm wanes.

*Day 2 Exercise: Sign your name and put today's date on the following personal contract.*

*I AM COMMITTED TO LOVING MY BRAIN AND TREATING IT WITH RESPECT AND CARE.*

_____                    _____

SIGNATURE                                                                                       DATE

**3. Practice Tiny Habits: The smallest thing you can do today that will make the biggest difference.**

Tiny Habits are like baby steps—easy changes that will boost your sense of accomplishment and competence and, over time, evolve into bigger changes.

Each of these habits takes just a few minutes. They are anchored to something you do (or think or feel) every day—like getting out of bed, brushing your teeth, answering the phone, or driving your car.

The goal is for them to become automatic. The Tiny Habits format is:
"When I do X (or when X happens), I will do Y."

Example:   "When I drive, I will fasten my seatbelt to protect against head trauma."

Celebrate whenever you adopt a Tiny Habit. Celebrations can be simple—like a fist pump or saying "Attaboy/Attagirl" to yourself.

*Day 2 Exercise: Here are 12 tiny habits we developed for our patients.*
*Choose the ones that work best for you. Place a checkmark next to each Tiny Habit you try.*

| Tiny Habit Recipe # | Anchor | Tiny Behavior | Done |
|---|---|---|---|
| 1 | After my feet hit the floor | I will say, "It's going to be a great day"! | |
| 2 | After I get dressed for bed | I will reflect on one good thing that happened in my day. | |
| 3 | After I flush the toilet | I will think of one thing that I am grateful for. | |

| Tiny Habit Recipe # | Anchor | Tiny Behavior | Done |
|---|---|---|---|
| 4 | As I look at the menu to choose something to eat | I'll ask if the items I choose are good or bad for my brain. | |
| 5 | After I start to blame someone else | I will think of one thing that I could have done to improve the situation. | |
| 6 | After I brush my teeth | I will take my supplements. | |
| 7 | After my head hits the pillow | I will think of 3 things that went well that day. | |
| 8 | After an automatic negative thought (ANT) pops up | I will write it down and ask if it is true. | |
| 9 | After I get out of the shower | I will read my ONE PAGE MIRACLE. | |
| 10 | After I wash my hands | I will tense and relax my hands. | |
| 11 | After I pick up a new item at the grocery store | I will check the label for added sugar. | |
| 12 | After I start to argue | I will ask myself, "Is my behavior getting me what I want?" | |

**4. Similar to Tiny Habits ... Start with 1 Thing.**

Tana is a "jump the canyon" kind of person who likes to give 100% from the get-go. But many people aren't like that. Look at Nancy. She was 80 when she came to Amen Clinics from Oxford, England. She was obsessed, depressed, isolated, and had arthritis. She had read one of my books—*Change Your Brain, Change Your Life*—and said it was riveting, but it made her realize she had so much to change. So, she decided to start with just 1 thing.

That was the secret to her success.

- She started by drinking more water. Your brain is 80% water and being dehydrated by just 2% causes fatigue and focus problems. It helped!
- Then she started taking supplements.
- Then she started walking and dancing.
- Then she changed her diet.
- Then she engaged in new learning.
- Eventually, she taught her children and grandchildren how to love and care for their brains.

This simple tactic helps you cut big changes down to size. Don't aim for 110%. Take it 1 small step at a time and, once you're ready, another step after that. With every step you'll be gaining confidence and building momentum toward the BIG results you're looking for!

Nancy lost 70 pounds and improved her mood, motivation, sleep, and zest for life.

***Day 2 Exercise:** Write down 1 step you will take today to get started on your journey to transformation.*

| 1 STEP I WILL TAKE TODAY |
| --- |
|  |

## 5. Journal Daily

**Journaling is a critical part of our program.** Every day rate the most important symptoms you want to change on a scale of 1 – 10 (1 is very bad/10 is very good). This provides a basis for you to evaluate any changes you make.

***Day 2 Exercise:** Rate your symptoms on a daily basis during this course. Here is an example chart below.*

| Day | Anxiety | Mood | Energy | Stress | Motivation |
| --- | --- | --- | --- | --- | --- |
| Sunday |  |  |  |  |  |
| Monday |  |  |  |  |  |
| Tuesday |  |  |  |  |  |
| Wednesday |  |  |  |  |  |
| Thursday |  |  |  |  |  |
| Friday |  |  |  |  |  |
| Saturday |  |  |  |  |  |

**6. Be curious, not furious. Turn bad days into good data.**

Everyone messes up at some point, and so will you. Be curious about your behavior, not furious at your slip-ups or mistakes. Investigating setbacks can be extremely instructive if you take the time to really analyze them. It is the down times, the slip-ups, the setbacks, that teach you most of what you need to know if you embrace them and take time to learn from them. You have to turn bad days into useful information.

*Day 2 Exercise: Write about a mistake you made and what you learned from it.*

Example:

| MISTAKE | WHAT I LEARNED |
|---|---|
| I let my anxiety get out of control and ate too much sugar to feel better. | I have better tools to calm anxiety and will use one of them next time. |

| MISTAKE | WHAT I LEARNED |
|---|---|
|  |  |

**7. Change has its ups and downs.**

As I often tell my patients, the road to change is not a one-way street. Your journey will be like going up and down a staircase. You'll go up several steps, feel like you've made progress, then go back down a few steps when difficult situations arise. You'll make several more steps of progress, then slip back a few, but usually not as many as before. Usually, the slope of progress is in an upward, positive direction.

Look at the following Change Diagram to know what to expect.

**CHANGE DIAGRAM**

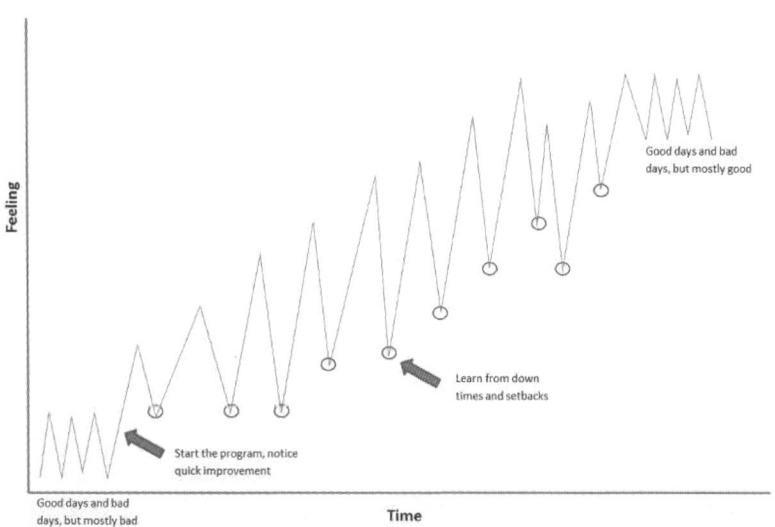

***Day 2 Exercise:** Write down one of your downtimes or setbacks and be curious about it. What can you learn from it?*

*Example:*

| SETBACK | WHAT I LEARNED |
|---|---|
| When I lost my job, I started falling back into old habits. | When things get stressful, I need to be extra careful about how I respond. |

| SETBACK | WHAT I LEARNED |
|---|---|
|  |  |

# DAY 3. KNOW YOUR BRAIN TYPE: BRAIN HEALTH ASSESSMENT

One of the most critical elements of overcoming anxiety, depression, trauma, and grief is healing your brain. The more you know about your brain, the better you can optimize it.

Not all brains are alike. Based on our brain imaging work at Amen Clinics, we have identified a total of 16 brain types (5 primary brain types and 11 combination brain types). Knowing your brain type helps you know more about how you interact with the world and what brain health/mental health risks you may face. Even more importantly, it can also help you understand how to optimize your specific brain to smooth out some of the rough edges.

**Day 3 Exercise: : Take the Brain Health Assessment at brainhealthassessment.com**

This assessment will reveal your Brain Type (based on our brain imaging work at Amen Clinics we have identified 16 brain types) and help you understand the health of your brain. It's easy.

• Click "Take the Quiz"

• Select "Let's Get Started!"

The assessment will take approximately 5 minutes and your results will be made available by download or email.

Write your Brain Type below.

**MY BRAIN TYPE**

**BRAIN TYPE # \_\_\_\_\_**

_____

# DAY 4. KNOW YOUR BRIGHT MINDS RISK FACTORS

To have a healthy mind, you must first have a healthy brain. To do that you must prevent or treat the 11 major BRIGHT MINDS risk factors that damage the brain and steal your mind. The BRIGHT MINDS Risk Factor Assessment will help you identify your risk factors and then you can use the BRIGHT MINDS Risk Factors & Strategies chart to learn how to prevent or treat your risk factors.

*Day 4 Exercise: In the chart below, circle your risk factors and take note of the strategies that can help you eliminate that risk.*

### BRIGHT MINDS RISK FACTORS & STRATEGIES

| Factors | Risks | Strategies |
|---|---|---|
| **B**lood Flow | Stroke, hypertension, or any form of heart disease<br>Little to no exercise | Get treatment early<br>Start prevention strategies<br>Eat foods such as beets and cayenne pepper<br>Take supplements such as Ginkgo<br>Exercise (30 minutes a day) |
| **R**etirement/Aging | No new learning<br>In a job that does not require new learning<br>Loneliness<br>Social isolation | Make new learning part of your everyday life<br>Take a class<br>Get involved with your family or church<br>Volunteer to help others |
| **I**nflammation | Standard American Diet (SAD) filled with fast and processed food<br>Low omega-3 levels<br>High C-reactive protein (CRP) levels (blood test) | Eat an anti-inflammatory diet<br>Increase dietary omega-3 fatty acids<br>Take supplements, such as fish oil, probiotics, and curcumins |
| **G**enetics | Family history of mental health issues or dementia | If you have a family history of mental health issues or dementia in your family, it is critical to be serious about brain health as soon as possible<br>Get screened early |

| Factors | Risks | Strategies |
|---|---|---|
| **H**ead Trauma/ Concussions | Head injury even without loss of consciousness | Protect your head<br>Wear a helmet when biking, skiing, etc.<br>Refrain from contact sports<br>Wear your seat belt<br>Avoid climbing ladders<br>Hold handrails when going up or down stairs<br>Never text while walking or driving |
| **T**oxins | Smoking<br>Drugs<br>Alcohol<br>Mold<br>Pesticides<br>Toxic products | Avoid toxic exposure and support the 4 organs of detoxification:<br><br>- *Kidneys – drink more water*<br>- *Gut – eat more fiber and choose organic foods*<br>- *Liver – quit smoking and drugs, limit alcohol, eat brassicas (cabbage, broccoli, cauliflower, and Brussels sprouts)*<br>- *Skin – sweat with exercise and take saunas*<br><br>Get tested for mold exposure<br><br>Download the 'Think Dirty' app to scan your personal products to know if they're toxic |
| **M**ind-Storms | Seizures or history of seizures<br>Frequent complaints that things look, sound, taste, feel, or smell "funny"<br>Visual or auditory changes | Ketogenic diet<br>NeuroFeedback<br>Stress-relief techniques<br>Avoid video games and flashing lights<br>Eliminate sugary foods, food dyes, or and food preservatives |
| **I**mmunity/Infections | Low vitamin D level<br>Lyme disease<br>Asthma<br>Autoimmune disorders, such as multiple sclerosis | Boost vitamin D intake and eat onions, mushrooms, and garlic<br>Work with an integrative or functional medicine doctor who can properly diagnose and treat you |
| **N**eurohormone Deficiencies | Abnormal thyroid, DHEA, testosterone, estrogen, and progesterone in females | Test and optimize your hormones |

| Factors | Risks | Strategies |
|---|---|---|
| **D**iabesity | Diabetes (high fasting blood sugar)<br>Being overweight or obese (high BMI) | Eliminate sugar<br>Follow BRIGHT MINDS diet<br>Eat calorie-smart |
| **S**leep Problems | Insomnia<br>Sleep apnea | Target 7-8 hours<br>Get an evaluation for sleep apnea if you snore<br>Practice good sleep hygiene |

# DAY 5. KNOW YOUR IMPORTANT NUMBERS

Maintaining your overall health is important to your brain health and your ability to keep your dragons under control. Below are 10 important numbers everyone should know and optimize.

### 1. Body Mass Index (BMI)
The BMI tells you the health of your weight compared to your height. Your doctor can calculate it, or you can easily find a BMI calculator online.

- Normal: 18.5-24.9
- Overweight: 25-30
- Obese: >30

### 2. Waist-to-Height Ratio

This is another way to measure the health of your weight. Divide your waist size by your height in inches. Note: You have to measure your waist size at your belly button! Do not guess or go by your pants size. Sizes can vary depending on the clothing manufacturer and many people have bellies that hang over their waistbands.

**Women**
Ratio less than .35: underweight
Ratio .35 to .42: extremely slim
Ratio .42 to .49: healthy
Ratio .49 to .54: overweight
Ratio .54 to .58: seriously overweight
Ratio over .58: highly obese

**Men**
Ratio less than .35: underweight
Ratio .35 to .43: extremely slim
Ratio .43 to .53: healthy
Ratio .53 to .58: overweight
Ratio .58 to .63: seriously overweight
Ratio over .63: highly obese

### 3. Blood Pressure

High blood pressure is associated with lower overall brain function.
Systolic (high number) _____
Diastolic (low number) _____

Check your blood pressure or have your doctor check it on a regular basis. If your blood pressure is high, make sure to take it seriously. Some behaviors that can help lower blood pressure include losing weight, daily exercise, fish oil and, if needed, medication.
- Optimal: Systolic 90-120, Diastolic 60-80
- Stage 1 Hypertension: Systolic 130-139, Diastolic 80-89
- Stage 2 Hypertension: Systolic ≥ 140, Diastolic ≥ 90
- Hypotension (too low can also be a problem): Systolic < 90, Diastolic < 60

**4. Vitamin D Level**

Low levels of vitamin D have been associated with obesity, depression, cognitive impairment, heart disease, and many other diseases. Have your physician check your 25-hydroxy vitamin D level, and if it is low get more sunshine and/or take a vitamin D supplement.

Low < 30 ng/dL
Optimal between 50-100 ng/dL

**5. Thyroid**

Having low thyroid levels decreases overall brain activity, which can impair your thinking, judgment, and self-control, and make it very hard for you to lose weight.

> _____ TSH (according to the American Association of Clinical Endocrinologists, anything over 3.0 is abnormal and needs further investigation)
> _____ Free T3 (see the normal ranges for the individual laboratory you use)
> _____ Free T4 (see the normal ranges for the individual laboratory you use)

There is no one perfect way, no one symptom or test result, that will properly diagnose low thyroid function or hypothyroidism. The key is to look at your symptoms and your blood tests, and then decide. Doctors typically diagnose thyroid problems by testing your TSH levels and sometimes your T3 and T4 levels.

**6. C-Reactive Protein (CRP)**

This measures the general level of inflammation but does not tell you where it is from.

Healthy: 0.0-1.0 mg/dL

The most common reason for an elevated C-reactive protein is metabolic syndrome or insulin resistance. The second most common is some sort of reaction to food—either a sensitivity, a true allergy, or an autoimmune reaction as occurs with gluten. It can also indicate hidden infections.

**7. Hemoglobin A1C (HbA1C)**

This test shows your average blood sugar levels over the past 2-3 months and is used to diagnose diabetes and prediabetes.

- Normal (for someone without diabetes): 4.0-5.6%
- Optimal: 5.3% or less
- Prediabetes: 5.7-6.4%

## 8. Lipid Panel

Make sure your doctor checks your total cholesterol level as well as your HDL (good cholesterol), LDL (bad cholesterol), and triglycerides (a form of fat). Normal levels are:

- Total cholesterol (135-200 mg/dL; below 160 has been associated with depression, suicide, homicide, and death from all causes, so 160-200 mg/dL is optimal)
- HDL (≥ 60 mg/dL)
- LDL (<100 mg/dL)
- Triglycerides (<100 mg/dL)

If your lipids are off, make sure to get your diet under control, take a high-quality fish oil supplement, and exercise. Of course, you should see your healthcare provider. Also, knowing the particle size of LDL cholesterol is very important. Large particles are less toxic than smaller particle size.

## 9. Testosterone

Low levels of testosterone, for men or women, are associated with low energy, heart disease, obesity, depression, and Alzheimer's disease.

Normal levels for adult males:
> Testosterone Total Male (280-800 ng/dL)—Optimal is 500-800 ng/dL
> Testosterone Free Male (7.2-24 picogram (pg)/mL)—Optimal is 12-24 pg/mL

Normal levels for adult females:
> Testosterone Total Female (6-82 ng/dL)—Optimal is 40-82 ng/dL
> Testosterone Free Female (0.0-2.2 pg/mL)—Optimal is 1.0-2.2 pg/mL

## 10. Ferritin

Ferritin is a measure of iron stores and increases with inflammation and insulin resistance.

Optimal: 30-100 ng/mL

Low levels are associated with anemia, restless leg syndrome, ADD, and low motivation and energy. Women often have lower iron stores than men because of menstruation. Some theorize that this is one of the reasons that women tend to live longer than men. If your level is low, consider taking iron. If it is high, donating blood may help.

***Day 5 Exercise:*** *Make an appointment and take the following Suggested Lab Panel to your healthcare provider. If you aren't able to get an appointment right away or it takes time to get your results, that's okay. You can continue with this 6-week program and use the information from your results when you get them.*

**NUTRITION**

Date: _____

Patient Name: _____

*General:*

- ☐ CBC (Complete Blood Count)
- ☐ Comprehensive Metabolic Panel
- ☐ DHEA-S
- ☐ Ferritin
- ☐ Free T3
- ☐ Free T4
- ☐ Hemoglobin A1C
- ☐ Homocysteine
- ☐ Hs-C-Reactive Protein (CRP)
- ☐ Insulin
- ☐ Lipid Panel
- ☐ Testosterone, Total and Free
- ☐ TSH (Thyroid Stimulating Hormone)
- ☐ Vitamin B12
- ☐ Vitamin D, 25-OH

# DAY 6. KNOW YOUR DRAGONS

To tame your dragons, you first need to recognize which hidden Dragons from the Past are impacting your life.

*Day 6 Exercise: Take the Know Your Dragons Questionnaire.*

## Know Your Dragons Questionnaire

Check any of the following that apply to you or your ancestors. Checking 2 or more in any one area indicates you likely have this Dragon. You can also take the quiz at knowyourdragons.com.

**Abandoned, Invisible, or Insignificant Dragons**

1. Do you often feel overlooked or unimportant?
2. Are you often lonely?
3. Do you crave attention or praise from others?
4. While you were growing up were your mother or father emotionally or physically unavailable to you? Were they absent or neglectful?
5. Growing up did you often feel small, invisible, or insignificant?

**Inferior or Flawed Dragons**

6. Did you grow up feeling "less than" others (ability, looks, achievement, or relationships)?
7. Were you often criticized by parents or other authority figures?
8. Do you frequently compare yourself to others in a negative way?
9. Do you feel like you must be perfect to be any good at all?
10. When you look in the mirror is your first tendency to notice what is wrong about yourself?

**Anxious Dragons**

11. Did you have a stressful or unpredictable childhood?
12. Do you have frequent feelings of nervousness, anxiety, or panic?
13. Do you tend to predict the worst or see the future with fear?
14. Are you sensitive to rejection or have a fear of being judged by others?
15. Do you tend to avoid conflict at all costs?

**Wounded Dragons**

16. Have you experienced significant emotional trauma in the past, such as bullying or physical, emotional, or sexual abuse?

17. Have you experienced intense periods of stress, such as being taken into foster care, or being in a fire, flood, or assault?

18. Do you have recurrent and upsetting thoughts of a past traumatic event (pandemic lockdown, molestation, accident, fire, etc.)?

19. Do you have marked physical responses to events that remind you of a past upsetting event (such as sweating when getting in a car if you had been in a car accident)?

20. Do you avoid situations that cause you to remember an upsetting event?

**Should and Shaming Dragons**

21. Were you raised in a culture of shame or guilt, where people tried to control you by making you feel bad?

22. Were you often humiliated, embarrassed, belittled, judged, or criticized?

23. Do you want to hide, withdraw, or engage in self-harmful behaviors in secret?

24. Do you routinely feel like guilt is motivating your actions and prompting you to do things that don't fit your wants or goals?

25. Do you often think in words like should, must, ought, and have-to?

**Special, Spoiled, or Entitled Dragons**

26. Did you have parents or caregivers who never said no to you?

27. Do you tend to lack empathy for others?

28. Do you get angry or rude if you don't get your way?

29. Do you feel like others should do things for you?

30. Do you often say, "You owe me …" "I deserve …" or "It's their fault …"

**Responsible Dragons**

31. Did you ever feel powerless to help someone you loved who was suffering?

32. Does helping others make you feel significant?

33. If something bad happened to a loved one (illness, accident, etc.), did you think it was your fault?

34. Do you feel it's your duty to help others?

35. Do you tend to take on too much responsibility?

**Angry Dragons**

36. While growing up were you hurt, shamed, bullied, abused, or disappointed by others?

37. Do you experience frequent anger or irritability?

38. Do you get easily frustrated and take it out on others?

39. Have people ever told you that are rude or inconsiderate?

40. Do you tend to purposely ignore others or act in a belittling or condescending way when upset?

**Judgmental Dragons**

41. Growing up did you perceive life was unfair?

42. Do you feel a need to correct others when they are wrong?

43. Do you tend to be critical of others?

44. Do you tend to tell others what they should think or feel?

45. Do you say things like, "If I was king or queen the world would be a better place?"

**Death Dragons**

46. Early in life did someone you care about become seriously ill or die?

47. Does death preoccupy your thoughts?

48. Do you have a pervading sense of doom?

49. Are you afraid of aging or losing your youth?

50. Do you worry about yourself or someone you love getting sick?

**Grief and Loss Dragons**

51. Have you lost someone important to you that you continue to think about? (such as through death, separation, or divorce; breakup of a love interest, close friend, or peer group; having a partner with dementia; or empty nest syndrome).

52. Have you lost something important? (such as your health, job, finances)

53. Have you lost an attachment to ideas or what could have been? (identity, success, having a healthy child – when yours has a disability)

54. Do you have anxiety or depression that still persists after a loss?

55. Do you find it hard to let go of what might have been?

**Hopeless or Helpless Dragons**

56. Do you often feel hopeless, helpless, or worthless?

57. Do you often feel sad or depressed?

58. Do you feel powerless to change how you feel?

59. Do your thoughts tend to be negative?

60. Do you often feel life is not worth living?

**Ancestral Dragons**

61. Did your parents, grandparents, or other ancestors experience significant emotional trauma or loss?

62. Did any of your ancestors die early (illness, accident, violence, suicide)?

63. Were any of your ancestors the victim, witness, perpetrator, or the falsely accused of a serious crime?

64. Were any of your ancestors abandoned by, or separated from their family?

65. Do have seemingly unfounded fears, anxiety, or behaviors that make little to no sense to you?

## MY DRAGONS

In the chart below, circle each of your dragons based on the questionnaire. On upcoming days of this program you'll discover more about their origins, triggers, and reactions, as well as strategies to tame your dragons so you can overcome anxiety, depression, trauma, and grief.

| Abandoned, Invisible, or Insignificant | Responsible | Judgmental | Ancestral |
|---|---|---|---|
| Inferior or Flawed | Special, Spoiled, or Entitled | Grief and Loss | Anxious |
| Angry | Death | Wounded | Should and Shaming |
| Hopeless or Helpless | | | |

SIX WEEKS TO OVERCOME ANXIETY, DEPRESSION, TRAUMA, AND GRIEF

# DAY 7. KNOW YOUR ANTS

Today, you'll learn one of the most powerful tools to change your life. Your brain is always listening to the ANTs (automatic negative thoughts) that fuel your dragons, steal your happiness, and ruin your life. To tame your dragons and overcome anxiety, depression, trauma, and grief, you must eliminate the ANTs with our ANT-killing process. If you do this diligently, you'll stop feeding your dragons, end self-defeating thoughts, and be more in control of your emotions and destiny.

*Day 7 Exercise: Circle the ANT Species that are infesting your brain and the types of thoughts you often have.*

**9 TYPES OF ANT SPECIES AND THE DRAGONS THEY FUEL**

| ANT SPECIES | TYPES OF THOUGHTS | DRAGONS THEY FUEL |
|---|---|---|
| All or Nothing | Thinking that things are either all good or all bad | Judgmental |
| Less Than | When you compare and see yourself less than others | Abandoned, Invisible, or Insignificant Inferior or Flawed |
| Just the Bad | Seeing only the bad in a situation | Wounded, Ancestral, Hopeless or Helpless, Death |
| Guilt Beating | Thinking in words like should, must, ought, or have to | Should and Shaming |
| Labeling | Attaching a negative label to yourself or someone else | Should and Shaming, Judgmental |
| Fortune Telling | Predicting the worst possible outcome for a situation with little or no evidence for it | Anxious, Wounded Hopeless or Helpless |
| Mind Reading | Believing you know what other people are thinking even though they haven't told you | Abandoned, Invisible, or Insignificant Inferior or Flawed Anxious |
| If Only and I'll Be Happy When | When you argue with the past and long for the future | Inferior or Flawed Anxious Wounded Should and Shaming Judgmental Grief and Loss |
| Blaming | Blaming someone or something else for your problems | Special, Spoiled, or Entitled |

## Learn the ANT Killing Process

Whenever you feel sad, mad, nervous or out of control, write down your ANTs and identify which type it is (there may be more than one type). Then ask yourself 5 simple questions. These questions are life-changing. When you answer them, there are no right or wrong answers; they are just questions to open your mind to alternative possibilities. Meditate on each answer to see how they make you feel. Ask if your stressful thoughts make your life better or worse. This powerful ANT–killing process is based on the work of psychiatrist Aaron Beck, who pioneered Cognitive Behavior Therapy, and author Byron Katie.

**ANT:** _____

**ANT Type(s):** _____

### 5 Questions

*Is it true?*
**Sometimes this first question will stop the ANT because you already know it's not true. Sometimes your answer will be "I don't know." If you don't know, then do not act like the negative thought is true. Sometimes you may think or feel that the negative thought it true, but that is why the second question is so important**

*Is it absolutely true with 100% certainty?*

*How do I feel when I believe this thought?*

*How would I feel if I couldn't have this thought?*

*Turn the thought around to its exact opposite, and then ask if the opposite of the thought is true or even truer than the original thought.*

*Use this turnaround as a meditation.*

*Example:*

Like so many people during the pandemic, Tana experienced some feelings of anxiety, and at one point, she said: "Nothing will ever be normal again." Here's how Tana answered the 5 questions to work on that thought.

**ANT:** *"Nothing will ever be normal again."*

**ANT Type:** *Fortune Telling*

## 5 Questions

*Is it true?*
**Yes**

*Is it absolutely true with 100% certainty?*
**No, some things may go back to normal, but there may be a new normal for other things.**

*How do I feel when I believe this thought?*
**Anxious, powerless, hopeless, out of control.**

*How would I feel if I couldn't have this thought?*
**Relieved, in control, like my usual self.**

*Turn the thought around to its exact opposite:*
**Some things will be normal again.**

*Any evidence that's true?*
**Yes, some things are already starting to return to how they were before the pandemic.**

*The thought to meditate on: Some things will be normal again.*

**Day 7 Exercise: Challenge one of your ANTs. Write down a negative thought and ask yourself the 5 questions.**

ANT: _____

ANT Type (s): _____

Is it true? ____

Is it absolutely true with 100% certainty? ____

How do I feel when I believe this thought?

_____

_____

How would I feel if I couldn't have this thought?

_____

_____

**Turn the thought around to its exact opposite, and then ask if the opposite of the thought is true or even truer than the original thought.**

_____

_____

**Then use this turnaround as a meditation.**

_____

# Week 2

# DAY 8. KNOW YOUR ONE PAGE MIRACLE AND MOTIVATION TO BE WELL

**Day 8. Know Your One Page Miracle (OPM) and Motivation to Be Well**

Tell your brain what you want and then your brain will help you match your behavior to get it! Your brain helps you make happen what it sees. When you focus on negativity, you will feel depressed. If you focus on fear you are likely to feel anxious. If you focus on achieving your goals, you are much more likely to achieve your goals.

Too many people are thrown around by the whims of the day, rather than using their brains to plan their lives and follow through on their goals.

The most powerful yet simple motivation exercise that we've designed is called the ONE PAGE MIRACLE (OPM). It will help guide your thoughts, words, and actions. It is called the ONE PAGE MIRACLE because we've seen this exercise quickly focus and change many people's lives.

*Day 8 Exercise: Create a OPM. Here are the steps:*

1. On the form provided in this workbook, write down what you want (not what you don't want) in the major areas of your life, including your relationships, work, money, and self (physical, emotional, and spiritual health).

2. Place it somewhere you can see it every day, such as on the refrigerator or bathroom mirror.

3. Ask yourself every day, "Is MY behavior today getting me what I want? DOES IT FIT?" This will help you focus your thoughts and actions on your goals throughout the day.

**ONE PAGE MIRACLE**

**What do I want in my relationships with my:**

Partner _____
_____
Children _____
_____
Extended family _____
_____
Friends _____

Clients _____

**What do I want in my work?** _____

**What do I want in my finances?** _____

**What do I want for myself in these areas:**

Physical _____

Emotional _____

Spiritual _____

***Day 8 Exercise: Fork in the Road***

1. Imagine yourself coming to a fork in the road.

2. Down one road, you're heading down a path to destruction, continuing your bad habits. At the end of that road, you can see how anxious, unhappy, and miserable you'll be. I want you to dwell on this to see if that is what you really want.

3. Now take the other road—the road to a commitment to good habits. At the end of this road, you can see your happiness increasing, anxiety decreasing, and outlook getting brighter.

4. Before you take any action, ask yourself one simple question: Does it fit? Does your behavior keep you on the road to happiness and peace? Or is it putting you on the road to despair?

_____

*Day 8 Exercise: Anchor Images*

Did you know that 50% of the brain is dedicated to vision? Visual cues are powerful reminders of motivation. Pick 4-5 images you can use to remind yourself every day why you must get healthy.

**Examples of Tana's anchor images:**

Husband Daniel

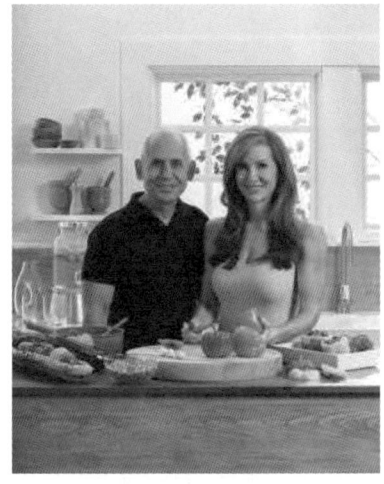

Daughter Chloe

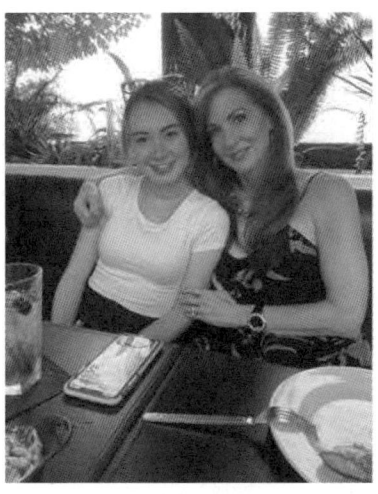

Nieces Alizé and Amelie and Chloe

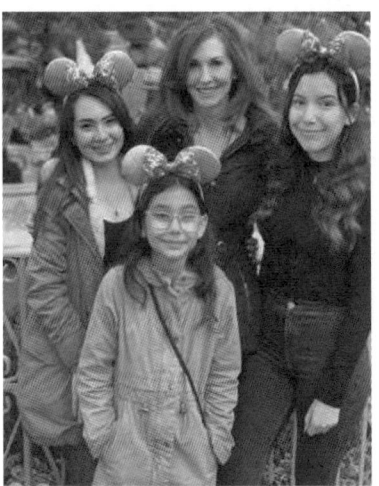

Dog Aslan

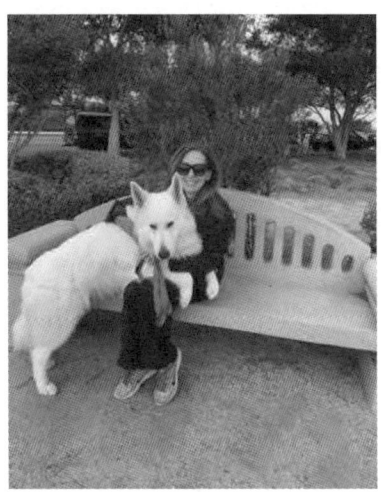

SIX WEEKS TO OVERCOME ANXIETY, DEPRESSION, TRAUMA, AND GRIEF

# MY ANCHOR IMAGES

*Place 4-5 photos on this page and put it somewhere you can see it every day:*

# DAY 9. 6 FEELING BETTER FAST TECHNIQUES

Today, you'll discover 6 ways to make yourself feel better fast when you're feeling anxious, depressed, stressed, or overwhelmed. They are very simple to do, they work quickly, and they have no downsides.

**1. Havening**

Havening is a very simple strategy—so easy even children can do it—you can use to calm yourself and wash away anxiousness or anger. It stimulates both sides of the brain and creates calming brainwaves in the emotional centers of the brain.

***Day 9 Exercise: Practice havening whenever you're upset, stressed, or anxious.***

1. Cross your arms and put each hand on the opposite shoulder.
2. Gently stroke down.
3. While you're stroking down, say, "I am safe, I am here, this is now."
4. Repeat for 30-60 seconds.

**2. Diaphragmatic Breathing (3 + 6 X 10).**

When you're feeling anxious or angry, your breathing becomes shallow and fast. This causes a change in oxygen in your blood, making you more anxious. It becomes a vicious cycle, causing irritability, impulsiveness, confusion, and bad decision-making.

Learning to direct and control your breathing has immediate benefits. It calms the brain's amygdala (the brain's fear centers), counteracts the body's stress response, relaxes muscles, warms hands, and regulates heart rhythms. This simple diaphragmatic breathing exercise can help calm you almost immediately.

***Day 9 Exercise: Practice 3 + 6 X 10 breathing to calm yourself***

1. Inhale for 3 seconds through your nose.
2. Hold for 1 second.
3. Exhale for 6 seconds (twice as long as inhale).
4. Hold for 1 second.
5. Repeat 10 times. This will take less than 2 minutes.

### 3. Hand Warming

Visualizing warmth, especially in your hands, is another tool to feel better fast and counteract the fight-or-flight response. I've found that when I teach patients to warm their hands, it calms down their bodies and minds just as effectively as prescription drugs. Hand warming elicits an immediate relaxation response by resetting your nervous system to counteract your stress response.

***Day 9 Exercise: Practice hand-warming for more relaxation.***

1. Close your eyes and hold your hands out, palms down, and visualize a campfire in front of you.

2. Focus. Think heat. You can hear the fire crackle, smell the aroma of fresh-cut wood burning, watch sparks fly and float up into the sky.

3. Now feel the soothing heat as it penetrates the surface of your skin and goes deep to warm your hands.

4. Picture this as you breathe deeply and count slowly to 20.

*Look at the list of hand-warming images below and choose the ones that work best for you. Place a checkmark next to the ones you will try.*

| 13 Potential Hand-Warming Images | Check Off √ |
|---|---|
| Holding someone's warm hand or touching their warm skin | |
| Appreciating someone else | |
| Putting your hands in warm sand at the beach | |
| Taking a hot bath or shower | |
| Sitting in a sauna | |
| Cuddling a baby | |
| Cuddling a warm, furry puppy or kitten | |
| Holding a warm cup of tea or sugar-free cocoa | |
| Holding your hands in front of a fire | |
| Wearing warm gloves | |
| Being wrapped in a warm towel | |
| Getting a massage with warm oil | |
| Holding a hot potato with warm gloves | |

## 4. Surround Yourself with Soothing Scents

Certain scents are known to have mood enhancing, calming, or stimulating effects. Use an essential oil diffuser and the following essential oils. **Place a checkmark next to the ones you will try.**

| Scent | Helpful for... | Check Off √ |
|---|---|---|
| Lavender | Anxiety<br>Grief<br>Memory<br>Pain Relief | |
| Chamomile | Anxiety | |
| Jasmine | Anxiety | |
| Ylang Ylang | Memory<br>Trauma<br>Anger | |
| Peppermint | Stimulating | |
| Eucalyptus | Stimulating<br>Focus | |

## 5. Create an Emotional Rescue Playlist

Music can soothe, inspire, improve your mood, and help you focus. In his powerful book, *The Secret Language of the Heart*, Barry Goldstein reviews the neuroscience properties of music and finds that it can:

- Stimulate emotional circuits in the brain
- Release oxytocin, the cuddle hormone
- Create peak emotions, which increase the amount of dopamine

***Day 9 Exercise: Create your own emotional rescue playlist to boost your mood quickly. Place a checkmark by the following suggested tunes you'll add to your emotional rescue playlist.***

**Without lyrics (words can be distracting):**

___ Sonata for Two Pianos in D Major (K. 448) – Mozart

___ Clair de Lune – Debussy

___ Adagio for Strings – Samuel Barber

___ Piano Sonata No. 17 in D Minor ("The Tempest") – Beethoven

___ Weightless – Marconi Union

___ Flotus – Flying Lotus

___ Lost in Thought – Jon Hopkins

___ Brain-enhancing music pieces specifically composed to enhance mood, memory, gratitude, creativity, energy, focus, motivation, and inspiration by Barry Goldstein (can be found at BrainMD.com).

**With lyrics:**

___ Good Vibrations – The Beach Boys

___ Don't Stop Me Now – Queen

___ Uptown Girl – Billy Joel

___ Dancing Queen – Abba

___ Eye of the Tiger – Survivor

___ I'm a Believer – The Monkeys

___ Girls Just Wanna Have Fun – Cyndi Lauper

___ Livin' on a Prayer – Bon Jovi

### 6. Loving Kindness Meditation

One of our favorite forms of meditation is called Loving Kindness Meditation (LKM), which is intended to develop feelings of goodwill and warmth toward others. It has been found to quickly increase positive emotions and decrease negative ones, decrease pain and migraine headaches, reduce symptoms of posttraumatic stress disorder and social prejudice, increase gray matter in the emotional processing areas of the brain, and boost social connectedness. Think of it as a way to soothe the hidden dragons inside you.

***Day 9 Exercise: Practice Loving Kindness Meditation.***

1. Sit in a comfortable and relaxed position and close your eyes.

2. Take 2-3 deep breaths, taking twice as long to exhale.

3. Let any worries or concerns drift away and feel your breath moving through the area around your heart.

4. As you sit, quietly or silently repeat the following or similar phrases:

    *May I be safe and secure*
    *May I be healthy and strong*
    *May I be happy and purposeful*
    *May I be at peace*

Let the intentions expressed in these phrases sink in as you repeat them. Allow the feelings to grow deeper. After a few repetitions, direct the phrases to someone you feel grateful for or someone who has helped you:

> *May you be safe and secure*
> *May you be healthy and strong*
> *May you be happy and purposeful*
> *May you be at peace*

Next, visualize someone you feel neutral about. Choose among people you neither like nor dislike and repeat the phrases.

Next, visualize someone you don't like or with whom you are having a hard time. Kids who are being teased or bullied at school often feel quite empowered when they send love to the people who are making them miserable.

Finally, direct the phrases toward everyone universally.

> *May all beings be safe and secure.*

You can do this for 10-30 minutes; it's up to you.

# DAY 10. SUPPLEMENT YOUR BRAIN

Today, you'll see how nutritional supplements can support your brain health and emotional well-being. We typically recommend 3 essential supplements to all of our patients because they are critical for optimal brain function: a multiple vitamin/mineral supplement, omega-3s, and vitamin D. In addition, it's a good idea to take targeted nutraceuticals to calm anxiousness, support moods, and promote emotional well-being.

*Day 10 Exercise: See the chart below for recommendations. You'll also receive recommendations for your brain type when you take the Brain Health Assessment (brainhealthassessment.com).*

| CATEGORY | TARGETED SUPPLEMENTS from BrainMD.com |
| --- | --- |
| ESSENTIALS | NeuroVite Plus<br>Omega-3 Power<br>Vitamin D |
| ANXIOUSNESS | GABA Calming<br>Everyday Stress Relief |
| LOW MOODS & NEGATIVITY | SAMe (s-adenosyl methionine)<br>Happy Saffron<br>Serotonin Mood Support<br>Methylfolate |
| FOCUS | Focus and Energy<br>Attention Support<br>Phosphatidylserine |
| CRAVINGS | Craving Control |
| CHRONIC STRESS | GABA Calming<br>Everyday Stress Relief |
| INSOMNIA | Put Me To Sleep<br>Restful Sleep<br>Magnesium Chewables<br>Serotonin Mood Support (if worrier) |

# DAY 11. BRAIN HEALTHY EATING

Whatever you put on the end of your fork matters! The foods you eat can increase feelings of anxiety and depression, decrease focus and attention, and increase the risk of dementia, or they can promote healthier moods, better focus, and a sharper mind. Today, you'll start with instructions on how to purge your pantry and you'll discover the 11 BRIGHT MINDS rules to follow that will help you feel the way you want to feel—less anxious, happier, and sharper.

**Purge Your Pantry**

The first thing you need to do is purge your pantry (as well as your refrigerator and your entire kitchen) and toss all of the foods that don't serve you and your family. Not having garbage food in the house helps prevent impulsive, mindless snacking as you change your eating patterns. It's easier to make 1 decision to get rid of it instead of 30 decisions over time not to eat it in a weak moment!

***Day 11 Exercise: Purge your pantry using the following list of items to toss! For more insight, watch us perform a step-by-step pantry purge in action on Tana's YouTube channel (https://www.youtube.com/watch?v=VqoWO0-RSAI).***

Here's a list of what to toss:

- The majority of processed foods. Most contain lots of unhealthy fat, sugar, corn syrup, artificial sweeteners, and other ingredients that you'll be avoiding. Beware of any products containing more than 5 ingredients or ingredients you can't pronounce.

- All foods that contain high-fructose corn syrup, sugar, artificial sweeteners, soy, trans fat, and hydrogenated and partially hydrogenated fat.

- The following cooking oils: vegetable oils, such as corn oil, safflower oil, canola oil, and soy-based oils.

- Cereal and other grain-based foods.

- Bread, pasta, and other foods that contain gluten.

- Fruit juice. Even if it's 100% fruit, juice causes unhealthy blood sugar spikes. Whenever fruit sugar is unwrapped from its fiber source, it can turn toxic in your liver.

- Foods that contain genetically modified ingredients.

- Foods that contain milk other dairy products. The exception is a bit of goat or sheep milk yogurt and cheese if you're not sensitive or allergic to them, or organic ghee.

- Cookies, cakes, candy, and other sweets.

- Condiments such as ketchup, barbecue sauce, and mustard (unless it's natural), which are usually packed with sugar, salt, and artificial ingredients and food coloring. Soy sauce contains gluten (usually), soy, and excessive sodium. Mustard that is gluten free and sugar free can stay. On rare occasions that you need soy sauce, choose organic, low-sodium tamari sauce, which is gluten free.

- Jams, jellies, and pancake syrup. They are pure sugar. Most "pancake" syrup contains no maple at all! It is high-fructose corn syrup and artificial flavoring.

**To optimize your brain and body, follow the 11 BRIGHT MINDS rules.**

**Rule #1: Go for "high-quality calories" (and not too many of them).**

Be mindful of your caloric intake and make sure you are consuming high-quality foods you love that love you back.

*Day 11 Exercise: Write down the low-quality foods—think high-fat, high-glycemic, pesticide-laden, processed foods—you currently eat. Which ones are you willing to ditch from your diet?*

_____    _____

_____    _____

_____    _____

_____    _____

**Rule #2: Water your brain.**

Drink half your weight in ounces of water a day to stay properly hydrated. Your brain is comprised of 80% water and being even mildly dehydrated can negatively impact your moods—making you feel more anxious, tense, depressed, or angry—in addition to sapping your energy levels and lowering your ability to concentrate.
Based on your weight, how many ounces of water do you need each day? _____

*Day 11 Exercise: What dehydrating beverages are you willing to give up now and replace with water?*

_____    _____    _____    _____

**Rule #3: Eat high-quality, lean protein throughout the day.**

As much as possible, make sure your protein sources (and the rest of your foods) are clean, which means organic, hormone-free, antibiotic-free, free range, and grass fed. The best sources of protein are:

- Eggs
- Fish (wild, not farmed)
- Lamb
- Turkey or chicken
- Raw nuts
- High-protein vegetables such as broccoli and spinach

*Day 11 Exercise: Write down protein sources you'll include in your diet.*

_____     _____

_____     _____

**Rule #4: Eat smart carbohydrates (low glycemic, high fiber).**

**Low Glycemic:** Generally speaking, you should eat foods on the lower end of the Glycemic Index (G.I.) to lower your blood glucose levels, decrease cravings, and help with weight loss. This should include vegetables, fruits, legumes, and nuts.

| *High G.I. foods I currently eat* | *I will replace with these low G.I. foods* |
|---|---|
| _____ | _____ |
| _____ | _____ |
| _____ | _____ |
| _____ | _____ |
| _____ | _____ |

**High Fiber:** These foods can help you lose weight! Dietary fiber helps regulate your sense of hunger, helps you feel fuller longer, and slows the absorption of food into your blood stream, which helps keep your blood sugar balanced.

Experts recommend adults eat 25 to 35 grams of fiber each day. Take a few minutes to calculate how much you have been getting on average each day, and if it falls below the recommended level, make a conscious effort to increase your fiber intake.

**Day 11 Exercise: Write down high-fiber foods you will add to your diet.**

_____     _____

_____     _____

**Rule #5: Focus your diet on healthy fats.**

Once the water is removed from it, your brain is about 60% fat, so fat is an important nutrient everyone needs. But we are talking about good fats, not unhealthy ones like trans fats.

*Which of these unhealthy fats are in your diet?*

☐ Trans fats: Also known as "hydrogenated" vegetable oils, trans fats are in many processed foods and baked goods

☐ Lard

☐ Marbled meat

☐ Full-fat dairy

☐ Fried foods

**Note:** You need to omit all of these completely from your diet. They are unnatural and unhealthy.

Replace unhealthy fats with healthy fats such as:

- Avocados
- Flax seeds
- Cold-water fish such as salmon
- Nuts
- Oils: coconut oil, grapeseed oil, olive oil

**Day 11 Exercise: Write down healthy fats you will add to your diet.**

_____     _____

_____     _____

**Rule #6: Eat from the rainbow.**

A healthy diet includes natural foods in a rainbow of colors.

*Day 11 Exercise: Write down your favorite fruits and vegetables that are:*

Yellow_____         Blue_____

Red _____           Purple_____

Green_____          Orange_____

**Rule #7: Cook with brain-healthy herbs and spices to boost your brain.**

Expand your repertoire of cooking using these brain healthy spices and herbs:

- Turmeric (found in curry) has been shown to decrease the brain plaques associated with Alzheimer's disease.

- Saffron can help with depression.

- Rosemary, thyme, and sage help boost memory.

- Cinnamon can help attention and blood sugar. It's also an antioxidant and an aphrodisiac.

- Garlic and oregano boost blood flow to the brain.

- Ginger, cayenne, and black pepper boost metabolism and have an aphrodisiac effect.

*Day 11 Exercise: Write down spices and herbs you will add to your diet.*

_____         _____

_____         _____

**Rule #8: Make sure your food is as clean as possible.**

Like rule #3 says, it's best to eat food that is: organic, hormone-free, antibiotic-free, free range, and grass fed. Furthermore, eliminate food additives, preservatives, artificial dyes, and sweeteners.

*Day 11 Exercise: Follow these guidelines the next time you go shopping.*

- *Read labels!*
- *If you can't pronounce it, don't eat it.*
- *If you don't know what is in something, don't eat it.*

**Rule #9: Check out food allergies.**

If you're having problems with your mood, energy, memory, weight, blood sugar, blood pressure, skin, or other health problems with no apparent cause identified by your doctor, you should consider eliminating wheat and any other gluten-containing grain or food, as well as dairy, soy, and corn.

*Day 11 Exercise: Consider an elimination diet (see Day 19) to see what foods might be causing you problems.*

**Rule #10: Eat for your Brain Type.**

Have you ever wondered why some people do well on high-protein diets while others feel irritable and can't stick with it? It depends on your brain type.

- **Balanced:** People with a balanced brain typically do well with a balanced diet.

- **Spontaneous:** People who are spontaneous or impulsive tend to do better on a high-protein diet.

- **Persistent:** People with the persistent brain type respond better to a diet that's higher in smart carbohydrates.

- **Sensitive:** People with are sensitive or sad typically do well on a balanced diet.

- **Cautious:** People who are cautious or anxious can eat a balanced diet.

*Day 11 Exercise: Check your Brain Type results (Day 3) to know more about eating for your type.*

**Rule #11: Find 25 foods you love that love you back.**

The secret to changing your diet is to find foods you love that love you back.

*Day 11 Exercise: Place a checkmark next to 25 of the brain healthy foods below that you love or that you will add to your diet.*

**Brain Healthy Fruits**
- ☐ Apples
- ☐ Avocados

- ☐ Berries (acai, blueberries, blackberries, goji berries, strawberries)
- ☐ Cherries
- ☐ Grapefruit
- ☐ Kiwi
- ☐ Oranges
- ☐ Peaches
- ☐ Plums
- ☐ Pomegranates

**Brain Healthy Veggies**
- ☐ Asparagus
- ☐ Beets
- ☐ Bok choy
- ☐ Broccoli
- ☐ Brussels sprouts
- ☐ Cabbage
- ☐ Cauliflower
- ☐ Celery
- ☐ Garlic
- ☐ Kale
- ☐ Leeks
- ☐ Onions
- ☐ Red bell peppers
- ☐ Seaweed
- ☐ Spinach

**Brain Healthy Nuts/Seeds**
Nuts (raw)
- ☐ Cacao
- ☐ Almonds
- ☐ Brazil nuts
- ☐ Cashews
- ☐ Walnuts

Seeds
- ☐ Chia
- ☐ Flax
- ☐ Hemp
- ☐ Sesame

### Roots
- [ ] Maca
- [ ] Shirataki noodles - wild
- [ ] Yam

### Brain Healthy Oils
- [ ] Avocado
- [ ] Coconut
- [ ] Macadamia
- [ ] Olive

### Brain Healthy Animal Products
(grass fed, hormone free, antibiotic free, free range, harvested humanely)
- [ ] Eggs
- [ ] Fish
- [ ] Lamb
- [ ] Chicken
- [ ] Turkey
- [ ] Beef

### Brain Healthy Beverages
- [ ] Water
- [ ] Coconut water
- [ ] Sparkling water with lemon and stevia
- [ ] Spa water with fruit

### Brain Healthy Sweeteners
- [ ] Stevia
- [ ] Xylitol
- [ ] Erythritol
- [ ] Honey – small doses

**Day 11 Exercise: Use the BrainFitLife app for brain healthy recipes from Tana. Visit TanaAmen.com for additional videos and resources on brain healthy eating, and order The Brain Warrior's Way Cookbook for more recipes and cooking tips.**

To overcome anxiety, depression, and other emotional hurts from your past, you need to nourish your brain without fueling your dragons.

***Day 11 Exercise: Using the chart below, circle the foods that feed your brain to lower your symptoms that you will add to your diet. Consider eliminating or limiting the items that will starve your dragons.***

| SYMPTOMS | FEED YOUR BRAIN | STARVE YOUR DRAGONS |
|---|---|---|
| ANXIETY | **GABA-rich foods:** Broccoli, almonds, walnuts, lentils, bananas, beef liver, brown rice, halibut, gluten-free whole oats, oranges, rice bran, and spinach<br><br>**Magnesium–rich foods:** Pumpkin and sunflower seeds, almonds, spinach, Swiss chard, sesame seeds, beet greens, summer squash, quinoa, black beans, and cashews<br><br>**Omega-3-rich foods:** Flaxseeds, walnuts, salmon, sardines, beef, shrimp, walnut oil, chia seeds, avocados, and avocado oil<br><br>**Probiotic-rich foods:** Brined vegetables, kimchi, sauerkraut, kefir, miso soup, pickles, spirulina, chlorella, and kombucha tea<br><br>**Drink green tea** for L-theanine | **LIMIT**<br>Caffeine, Alcohol, Sugar |
| MOOD | **Fruits and vegetables:** Eat up to 8 servings a day to boost levels of happiness; tomatoes have been shown to lift mood<br><br>**Serotonin–rich foods:** Combine tryptophan-containing foods (eggs, turkey, seafood, chickpeas, nuts, and seeds) with healthy carbohydrates like sweet potatoes and quinoa to drive insulin into the brain<br><br>**Omega-3-rich foods:** Flaxseeds, walnuts, salmon, sardines, beef, shrimp, walnut oil, chia seeds, avocados, and avocado oil<br><br>**Probiotic-rich foods:** Brined vegetables, kimchi, sauerkraut, kefir, miso soup, pickles, spirulina, chlorella, and kombucha tea<br><br>**Prebiotic-rich foods:** : Dandelion greens, psyllium, artichokes, asparagus, beans, cabbage, raw garlic, onions, leeks, and root vegetables (carrots, jicama, beets, turnips, and more)<br><br>**MACA:** A root vegetable native to Peru | **LIMIT** Simple carbs, such as:<br>Bread<br>Rice<br>Pasta<br>Potatoes |
| TRAUMA & GRIEF | **Serotonin-rich foods:** Eggs, turkey, seafood, chickpeas, nuts and seeds, sweet potatoes, quinoa, and dark chocolate (only in small amounts)<br><br>**GABA-rich foods:** Broccoli, almonds, walnuts, lentils, bananas, beef liver, brown rice, halibut, gluten-free whole oats, oranges, rice bran, and spinach<br><br>**Magnesium-rich foods:** Pumpkin and sunflower seeds, almonds, spinach, Swiss chard, sesame seeds, beet greens, summer squash, quinoa, black beans, and cashews<br><br>**Spices:** Saffron and turmeric | **LIMIT** Simple carbs, such as:<br>Bread<br>Rice<br>Pasta<br>Potatoes |

# BRIGHT MINDS STRATEGIES

To keep your brain healthy, or rescue it if it is headed for the dark place, you have to prevent or treat the 11 major risk factors that steal your mind.

For the next 11 days, we will take a deep dive into these risk factors and give you some simple suggestions on how to overcome them, which will translate into better emotional health, stronger resilience in difficult times, and more motivation to make the transformations you want.

# DAY 12. BRIGHT MINDS STRATEGY: BOOST BLOOD FLOW

Blood flow throughout your body brings oxygen and other nutrients to all your cells and carries away waste products. Surprisingly, the blood vessels that feed our brain cells age faster than those neurons, so keeping your brain healthy means taking care of your blood vessels. On SPECT, low blood flow is the #1 predictor of Alzheimer's disease. Low blood flow on SPECT has also been seen with depression, suicide, bipolar disorder, schizophrenia, ADD/ADHD, traumatic brain injury, hoarding, murder, substance abuse, seizure activity, and more.

**YOUR PERSONAL RISK CHECKLIST: WHICH BLOOD FLOW RISK FACTORS DO YOU HAVE?**

If you are unsure whether you have any of the following risk factors, schedule a checkup with your healthcare provider, who will take your blood pressure, listen to your heart and order laboratory tests to assess the health of your blood vessels. You can always fill in this checklist when you have the results of your checkup and tests.

**CARDIOVASCULAR DISEASE**
- ☐ Atherosclerosis (hardening of the arteries)
- ☐ High LDL or total cholesterol
- ☐ Heart attack
- ☐ Atrial fibrillation
- ☐ Hypertension or prehypertension (Hypertensive: 140/90 or higher, Prehypertensive: 120/80 to 139/89)

**OTHER RISK FACTORS**
- ☐ Having a stroke or transient ischemic attack (TIA)
- ☐ Exercising less than twice a week and/or a slow walking speed. Ultimately, one of the most important reasons to exercise is that it keeps your blood vessels open and healthy
- ☐ Erectile dysfunction
- ☐ Episode(s) of a loss of oxygen to the brain (such as during sleep apnea, a near drowning, or a heart attack, when the heart stops beating)

**KEY BLOOD FLOW TESTS**
- ☐ Blood pressure: Both high and low blood pressure (less than 90/60) are a risk factor
- ☐ CBC (complete blood count)
- ☐ Lipid panel: Cholesterol levels that are too high or too low are bad for the brain

## STRATEGIES TO BOOST BLOOD FLOW
*Day 12 Exercise: Choose at least 1 of the following strategies to start today.*

1. **Avoid anything that hurts vascular health.** Examples include a sedentary lifestyle, caffeine and nicotine (both constrict blood flow to the brain and other organs), and dehydration

2. **Seek treatment for anything that damages your blood flow.** Be serious about addressing coronary artery disease, heart arrhythmias, pre-diabetes and diabetes, pre-hypertension and hypertension, insomnia, sleep apnea, and drug/alcohol abuse.

3. **Lose weight if your BMI is over 25.**

4. **Spend 10-20 minutes a day in deep prayer or meditation.** Both prayer and meditation have both been shown to improve blood flow to the brain. They are also wonderful stress management tools.

5. **Strengthen your blood brain barrier (BBB).** Eliminate gluten, dairy, and toxins, and treat any infections. Many of the supplements we recommend in the program also seem to help with the integrity of the BBB, such as vitamins folate, B6 and B12, vitamin D, acetyl-l-carnitine, curcumin, resveratrol, and omega-3 EPA and DHA.

6. **Adopt these natural strategies to keep your blood pressure healthy.** In addition to the other strategies on this list, the following will help keep your blood pressure healthy.

- Eat more plant-based foods
- Limit dairy
- Limit salt intake (about 1,500 mg a day is recommended; no more than 2,300 mg)
- Eat more foods high in magnesium (ex: pumpkin seeds) and potassium (ex: bamboo shoots, cabbage)
- Eat more foods with blood pressure–lowering effects, such as beet juice, broccoli, celery, garlic, chickpeas, spinach, and mushrooms
- Eliminate alcohol, caffeine, fruit juices, and sodas (including diet sodas)
- Drink water! People who drank at least 5 glasses of water a day have half the risk of hypertension as those who drink fewer than 2 glasses a day
- Donate blood
- Focus on getting 7 to 8 hours of sleep a night and if you have sleep apnea, get it assessed and treated
- Take supplements with research-based evidence to lower blood pressure: magnesium, potassium, CoQ 10, vitamins C and D, aged garlic, omega-3 fatty acids EPA and DHA

7. **Take medication if you need it**. At Amen Clinics we prefer to take a natural approach to health problems, but hypertension or excessively high cholesterol levels can become a health crisis if not managed properly, and the thoughtful use of medicine can be very helpful.

8. **Exercise!** Regular exercise helps to boost nitric oxide and keep blood vessels open and flexible. The following 4 types of exercise are great for your brain. Of course, you should check with your physician before starting any new exercise routines.

    > **Burst training.** This involves bursts of 30-60 seconds at go-for-broke intensity followed by a few minutes of lower-intensity exertion. I recommend you take a 30-45 minute walk every day. During the walk, take 4 or 5 one-minute periods to "burst" (walking or running as fast as you can), and walk at a normal pace between bursts. Short–burst training also helps raise endorphins, lift your mood, and make you feel more energized. When walking in everyday life, walk like you are late. Seniors who walked faster lived longer and had better executive function.

    > **Strength training.** The stronger you are as you age, the less likely you are to get Alzheimer's disease. Canadian researchers found that resistance training plays a role in preventing cognitive decline. It also helps with people who have mild cognitive impairment. We recommend 2 weight-lifting sessions a week—30-45 minutes each and a day or two apart—one for the lower body (abs, lower back and legs), the other for the upper body (arms, upper back and chest).

    > **Coordination activities.** Dancing, tennis, table tennis (the world's best brain sport) and similar types of exercise boost the activity in the cerebellum. While the cerebellum is only 10% of the brain's volume, it contains 50% of the brain's neurons. It's involved with both physical and thought coordination.

    > **Mindful exercise.** Yoga, tai chi and other mindful exercises have been found to reduce anxiety and depression and increase focus and energy. Although they don't offer the same BDNF-generating benefits as aerobic activity, these types of exercise can still boost your brain health.

9. **Hyperbaric oxygen therapy (HBOT).** HBOT is a simple, non-invasive, painless treatment that uses the power of oxygen to enhance the healing process and boost blood flow. Brain imaging studies using SPECT show that people who have had HBOT have marked improvement in blood flow to the brain.

## EAT MORE OF THESE HEART-HEALTHY FOODS AND SPICES

**Arginine-rich foods:** beets (and beet juice), pork, turkey, chicken, beef, salmon, halibut, trout, steel-cut oats, clams, watermelon, pistachios, walnuts, seeds, kale, spinach, celery, cabbage, and radishes

**Foods rich in vitamin B6, B12, and folate:** leafy greens, cabbage, bok choy, bell peppers, cauliflower, lentils, asparagus, garbanzo beans, spinach, broccoli, parsley, cauliflower, salmon, sardines, lamb, tuna, beef, and eggs

**Vitamin E–rich foods:** green leafy vegetables, almonds, hazelnuts, and sunflower seeds

**Magnesium-rich foods:** pumpkin and sunflower seeds, almonds, spinach, Swiss chard, sesame seeds, beet greens, summer squash, quinoa, black beans, and cashews

**Potassium-rich foods:** beet greens, Swiss chard, spinach, bok choy, beets, Brussels sprouts, broccoli, celery, cantaloupe, tomatoes, salmon, banana, onions, green peas, sweet potato, avocados, and lentils

**Fiber-rich foods:** green beans, peas, carrots, seeds, Brazil nuts

**Garlic:** considered a triple threat against infections due to its antibacterial, antiviral, and antifungal properties

**Vitamin C–rich foods:** oranges, tangerines, kiwifruit, berries, red and yellow bell peppers, dark green leafy vegetables (such as spinach and kale), broccoli, tomatoes, peas

**Polyphenol-rich foods/drinks:** green tea, coffee, blueberries

**Omega-3–rich foods:** flaxseeds, walnuts, salmon, sardines, beef, shrimp, walnut oil, chia seeds, avocado oil

**Maca:** a root vegetable native to Peru

**Spices:** cayenne pepper, ginger, garlic, turmeric, coriander and cardamom, cinnamon, rosemary, and bergamot

| SUPPLEMENT | RECOMMENDED DOSAGE | BRAINMD SOLUTIONS |
|---|---|---|
| Ginkgo biloba | 60-120 mg twice a day. Start at the lower dose for several weeks then increase to the higher dose to see which is best for you. | Brain and Memory Power Boost |
| Omega-3 fatty acids | 1.4 grams (or more) a day of a combination of EPA and DHA in about a 60/40 ratio | Omega-3 Power |

# DAY 13. BRIGHT MINDS STRATEGY: KEEP YOUR BRAIN YOUNG

Today, you'll discover that to help keep your brain young, you need to engage in lifelong learning. The best mental exercises involve acquiring new knowledge and doing things you haven't done before. New learning, such as a new hobby or game, establishes new connections, which maintains and improves other brain areas that you use less often.

The parts of your brain you use will grow, and the parts of your brain you don't use will atrophy or shrink. For example, if you only play Scrabble or only do the Sunday crossword puzzle, you won't get the full benefits you want. That's like going to work out and only doing right biceps curls and then leaving.

**YOUR PERSONAL RISK CHECKLIST**
**WHICH RETIREMENT/AGING RISK FACTORS DO YOU HAVE?**

If you are unsure whether you have any of the following risk factors, schedule a checkup with your healthcare provider, who can order laboratory tests for iron and other health measures related to aging. You can always fill in this checklist when you have the results of your checkup and tests.

- [ ] Age: I am ___ years
- [ ] Retirement/lack of new learning
- [ ] Social isolation
- [ ] Too much (or too little) iron
- [ ] Shortened telomeres (protective caps at the ends of chromosomes)

**KEY RETIREMENT/AGING TESTS**

While it is important to know all of your health numbers, the ones here are key to assessing how well you are aging. Be sure to have these tests done now.

- [ ] C-reactive protein (CRP): a measure of inflammation
- [ ] Fasting blood sugar: This blood test, along with Hemoglobin A1c, screens for prediabetes and diabetes
- [ ] Hemoglobin A1C (HbA1C)
- [ ] DHEA: Higher levels of this neurohormone, as well as testosterone, are associated with longevity
- [ ] Testosterone
- [ ] Ferritin (iron levels)
- [ ] Telomere length: Testing for CRP and HbA1C (see above) may be substituted for this test

## STRATEGIES TO KEEP YOUR BRAIN YOUNG
***Day 13 Exercise: Choose at least 1 of the following strategies to start today.***

1. Limit charred meats

2. Get your ferritin level checked

3. Donate blood if ferritin is too high

4. Try a daily 12-16 hour fast

5. Cloves as a potent antioxidant

6. Add acetylcholine-rich foods, such as shrimp

7. Stay connected, such as volunteering

8. Music training

9. Start a daily practice of learning something new

***Day 13 Exercise: Look at the graphic below for ideas to exercise different areas of your brain, then write down 1 new thing you'll learn today and the part of the brain it exercises.***

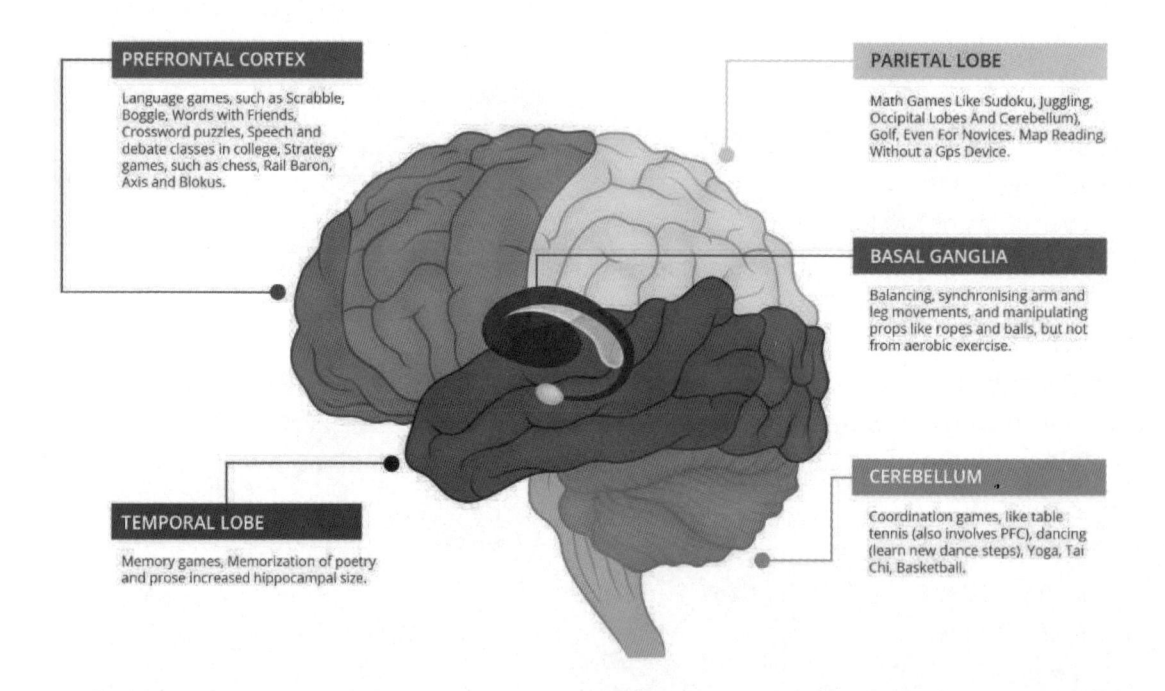

**PREFRONTAL CORTEX**
Language games, such as Scrabble, Boggle, Words with Friends, Crossword puzzles, Speech and debate classes in college, Strategy games, such as chess, Rail Baron, Axis and Blokus.

**PARIETAL LOBE**
Math Games Like Sudoku, Juggling, Occipital Lobes And Cerebellum), Golf, Even For Novices. Map Reading, Without a Gps Device.

**BASAL GANGLIA**
Balancing, synchronising arm and leg movements, and manipulating props like ropes and balls, but not from aerobic exercise.

**TEMPORAL LOBE**
Memory games, Memorization of poetry and prose increased hippocampal size.

**CEREBELLUM**
Coordination games, like table tennis (also involves PFC), dancing (learn new dance steps), Yoga, Tai Chi, Basketball.

| 1 NEW THING I'LL LEARN TODAY | WHAT PART OF MY BRAIN DOES IT EXERCISE? |
|---|---|
|  |  |

## NUTRACEUTICALS THAT SLOW AGING

| SUPPLEMENT | RECOMMENDED DOSAGE | BRAINMD SOLUTIONS |
|---|---|---|
| Phosphatidylserine | The typical adult dose is 100-300 mg a day | NeuroPS<br>Brain and Memory Power Boost |
| Huperzine A | The typical adult dose is 50-100 micrograms twice a day | Brain and Memory Power Boost |

## NUTRACEUTICALS THAT SLOW AGING

**Antioxidant-rich spices:** cloves, oregano, rosemary, thyme, cinnamon, turmeric, sage, garlic, ginger, fennel

**Antioxidant-rich foods:** acai fruit, parsley, cocoa powder, raspberries, walnuts, blueberries, artichokes, cranberries, kidney beans, blackberries, pomegranates, chocolate, olive and hemp oil (don't use either oil for cooking at high temperatures), dandelion greens, green tea

**Choline-rich foods:** to support acetylcholine and memory: shrimp, eggs, scallops, chicken, turkey, beef, cod, salmon, shiitake mushrooms, chickpeas, lentils, collard greens

**Allicin-rich foods:** raw, crushed garlic, onions, and shallots

**Polyphenol-rich foods/drinks:** green tea, coffee, blueberries

**Foods rich in vitamin B12 and folate:** leafy greens, cabbage, bok choy, bell peppers, cauliflower, lentils, asparagus, garbanzo beans, spinach, broccoli, parsley, cauliflower, salmon, sardines, lamb, tuna, beef, and eggs

# DAY 14. BRIGHT MINDS STRATEGY: QUELL INFLAMMATION AND IMPROVE GUT HEALTH

The word inflammation comes from the Latin inflammare, meaning "to set on fire." When you have high levels of inflammation in your body it is like having a low-level fire that destroys your organs and harms your brain and mind. It has been associated with a wide range of neurological and psychiatric illnesses, including:

- Depression
- Bipolar disorder
- OCD
- Schizophrenia
- Personality disorders
- Alzheimer's disease

**The Gut-Brain-Inflammation Connection**

The gut—your gastrointestinal tract (GI)—is often called the second brain because it is lined with so many nerve cells. This nervous tissue is in direct communication with the brain inside your skull. When the lining of your digestive tract becomes too permeable, it causes a condition known as leaky gut that is associated with inflammation.

Leaky gut is associated with brain health problems, including:

- Mood disorders
- Anxiety disorders
- ADD/ADHD
- Alzheimer's disease

**YOUR PERSONAL CHECKLIST**
**Which Inflammation Risk Factors Do You Have?**

While inflammation is your body's natural (and necessary) reaction to infection and injury, it's important to know what else can trigger inflammation and the conditions under which it can become chronic and harmful.

Check your inflammation risk factors:
- ☐ Cigarette smoking
- ☐ High blood sugar levels (See Day 21)
- ☐ Exposure to environmental toxins (see Day 17)
- ☐ Gum disease
- ☐ Leaky gut
- ☐ Low levels of omega-3 fatty acids

**Which Gut Health Risk Factors Do You Have?**

- ☐ Medications (antibiotics, oral contraceptives, proton pump inhibitors, steroids, NSAIDS)
- ☐ Low levels of omega-3 fatty acids
- ☐ Stress
- ☐ Sugar and high fructose corn syrup
- ☐ Artificial sweeteners
- ☐ Gluten
- ☐ Allergies to the environment or food
- ☐ Insomnia (especially among soldiers and those involved in shift work)
- ☐ Toxins (antimicrobial chemicals in soaps, pesticides, heavy metals)
- ☐ Intestinal infections (Helicobacter pylori, parasites, Candida)
- ☐ Low levels of vitamin D
- ☐ Radiation/chemotherapy
- ☐ Excessive high-intensity exercise
- ☐ Excessive alcohol

**KEY TESTS FOR INFLAMMATION**

While it is important to know all of your health numbers (See Day 5), the ones here are key to assessing whether or not inflammation is an issue for you. Be sure to have these blood tests done to assess your risk.

- ☐ C-reactive protein (CRP)
- ☐ Omega-3 Index (a measure of the omega-3 fatty acids EPA and DHA in red blood cells, which reflects brain levels of these fats)

**STRATEGIES TO CALM INFLAMMATION**

- ☐ Avoid smoking
- ☐ Stabilize blood sugar levels (Day 21)
- ☐ Eliminate toxins (Day 17)
- ☐ Get serious about flossing and gum health
- ☐ Repair leaky gut
- ☐ Eat prebiotic and probiotic foods for gut health (see below)

| SUPPLEMENT | RECOMMENDED DOSAGE | BRAINMD SOLUTIONS |
| --- | --- | --- |
| Omega-3 fatty acids | 1.4 grams (or more) a day of a combination of EPA and DHA in about a 60/40 ratio | Omega-3 Power<br>Omega-3 Power Squeeze |
| Curcumins | 500-2,000 mg a day of a highly bioavailable curcumin supplement | Brain Curcumins<br>Happy Saffron Plus |
| Probiotics | 3 billion live organisms a day, with both Lactobacillus and Bifidobacterium bacterial strains | ProBrainBiotics |

**EAT MORE OF THESE INFLAMMATION-FIGHTING FOODS AND SPICES**

*Day 14 Exercise: Choose at least 1 of the following anti-inflammatory foods.*

**Anti-inflammatory spices:** turmeric, cayenne, ginger, cloves, cinnamon, oregano, pumpkin pie spice, rosemary, sage, fennel

**Folate-rich foods:** spinach, dark leafy greens, asparagus, turnips, beets, mustard greens, brussels sprouts, lima beans, beef liver, root vegetables, kidney beans, white beans, salmon, avocado

**Omega-3-rich foods:** flaxseeds, walnuts, salmon, sardines, beef, shrimp, walnut oil, chia seeds, and avocado oil. (Animal sources provide EPA and DHA directly, but plant sources have to be converted, and some people's enzyme systems are poor at making this conversion.)

**Prebiotic-rich foods:** dandelion greens, asparagus, chia seeds, beans, cabbage, psyllium, artichokes, raw garlic, onions, leeks, root vegetables (sweet potatoes, yams, squash, jicama, beets, carrots, turnips)

**Probiotic-rich foods:** brined vegetables (not vinegar), kimchi, sauerkraut, kefir, miso soup, pickles, spirulina, chlorella, blue-green algae, kombucha

**PREBIOTIC FOODS I'LL ADD TO MY DIET**
- ☐ Apples
- ☐ Beans
- ☐ Cabbage
- ☐ Psyllium
- ☐ Artichokes
- ☐ Onions
- ☐ Leeks
- ☐ Asparagus
- ☐ Sweet Potatoes
- ☐ Yams
- ☐ Squash
- ☐ Jicama
- ☐ Beets
- ☐ Carrots
- ☐ Turnips

**PROBIOTIC FOODS I'LL ADD TO MY DIET**
- ☐ Kefir
- ☐ Kombucha
- ☐ Unsweetened Yogurt (Goat or Coconut)
- ☐ Kimchi
- ☐ Pickled Fruits
- ☐ Vegetables
- ☐ Sauerkraut

# Week 3

# DAY 15. BRIGHT MINDS STRATEGY: KNOW YOUR GENETICS

Brain health issues clearly run in families. If you have family members with issues, such as anxiety, depression, ADD/ADHD, OCD, bipolar disorder, schizophrenia, addictions, Alzheimer's disease, or Parkinson's, you have a higher risk of having them too. But having a genetic risk is not a death sentence. It should be a wakeup call for you to know your vulnerabilities and get serious about taking care of your brain.

**YOUR PERSONAL CHECKLIST**
**What Genetic Risk Factors Do You Have?**

☐ Family history of mental health problems, trauma, or memory issues
☐ Apolipoprotein E (APOE) gene—some variants of this gene are associated with increased risk of Alzheimer's disease

**KEY GENETIC TESTS**

☐ Family history of mental health problems, trauma, or memory issues
☐ Additional genetic testing (for other genes like presenilin genes 1 and 2 if family members have early-onset memory problems; ask your doctor about this)

**STRATEGIES TO ADDRESS YOUR GENETIC RISKS**
*Day 14 Exercise: Choose at least 1 of the following strategies to start today.*

☐ Believe your behavior can turn on or turn off the genes that increase your vulnerability for brain health and mental health issues.
☐ Get screened
      o Consider genetics testing to identify vulnerabilities
      o Cognitive and psychological testing
      o Questionnaires
      o Brain SPECT imaging
☐ Be serious about brain health and attack all of your BRIGHT MINDS risk factors
☐ Exercise aerobically, do balance exercises, and strengthen your muscles
☐ Protect your head from injury and concussions
☐ Learn more about your family history regarding mental health issues, trauma, or memory issues

**NUTRACEUTICALS TO SUPPORT BRAIN HEALTH**

| SUPPLEMENT | RECOMMENDED DOSAGE | BRAINMD SOLUTIONS |
|---|---|---|
| Multivitamin/Mineral | A high-quality, high-dose supplement | NeuroVite Plus |
| Omega-3 fatty acids | 1.4 grams (or more) a day of a combination of EPA and DHA in about a 60/40 ratio | Omega-3 Power<br>Omega-3 Power Squeeze |
| Vitamin D | 2,000 IU a day or more, depending on your level | Vitamin D3<br>NeuroVite Plus |

# DAY 16. BRIGHT MINDS STRATEGY: PROTECT YOUR BRAIN

Head trauma is more common than you might think. In the U.S., there are over 2 million new head injuries every year. At Amen Clinics, brain SPECT imaging shows that 40% of our patients have experienced a traumatic brain injury. Head trauma is a major risk factor for psychiatric illnesses, but few people know it because traditional psychiatry rarely looks at the brain. Research shows that head injuries increase the risk of:

- Anxiety
- Panic disorders
- Depression
- PTSD
- ADD/ADHD
- Psychosis
- Drug and alcohol abuse
- Memory problems and dementia
- Suicide
- Borderline and antisocial personality disorders
- Aggression

**YOUR PERSONAL CHECKLIST**
**Which Head Trauma Risk Factors Do You Have?**

Brain tissue is soft, like custard, and the bony skull that protects the brain has sharp ridges. As a result, anything that causes your brain to hit up against your skull can cause trauma—bruising, bleeding, lack of oxygen, damaged brain cells, and more. Here are some of the most common causes of head trauma. Put a checkmark next to the ones you have experienced.

- ☐ Family history of mental health problems, trauma, or memory issues
- ☐ Falls (down steps, off a ladder, out of bed, in the shower or bath, out of a tree, etc.)
- ☐ Motor vehicle accidents (car, motorcycle, truck, bicycle, ATV)
- ☐ Pedestrian-vehicle collisions
- ☐ Sports injuries (football, soccer, boxing, baseball, basketball, cycling, etc.)
- ☐ Combat injuries (including explosive blasts)
- ☐ Violence (gunshot wounds, domestic violence, an assault, etc.)

**KEY TESTS TO SCREEN FOR HEAD TRAUMA**

- ☐ Family history of mental health problems, trauma, or memory issues
- ☐ Consider getting a functional imaging study, such as SPECT or QEEG, if you're struggling with anxiety, depression, or other mental or cognitive issues

- ☐ Check out your sense of smell if you're having trouble smelling peanut butter, lemon, strawberry, or natural gas scents
- ☐ Omega-3 Index
- ☐ HbA1c and fasting blood sugar (high blood sugar levels can delay healing)
- ☐ Get your hormone levels tested, including thyroid, DHEA, and testosterone levels (head injuries often damage the master hormone gland, the pituitary, which can cause hormone deficiencies)

**STRATEGIES TO HELP HEAL THE BRAIN AFTER A HEAD INJURY**
*Day 16 Exercise: Choose at least 1 of the following strategies to start today.*

- ☐ **Avoid any future head injuries:**
    - o Avoid contact sports
    - o Avoid high-risk activities
    - o Don't climb trees or ladders or go on the roof
    - o Don't dive headfirst into any body of water
    - o Don't text while driving or walking
    - o Always wear a helmet when riding a bike or skiing
    - o Always wear your seatbelt in the car
- ☐ **Hyperbaric oxygen therapy (HBOT):** HBOT is a simple, non-invasive, painless treatment that uses the power of oxygen to enhance the healing process. Research shows it can be effective following a head injury.
- ☐ **Neurofeedback:** This is an interactive, non-invasive, medication-free treatment that helps strengthen and retrain the brain. It has been used successfully to improve brain function following a head injury.

**NUTRACEUTICALS TO SUPPORT BRAIN HEALING**

| SUPPLEMENT | RECOMMENDED DOSAGE | BRAINMD SOLUTIONS |
|---|---|---|
| Multivitamin/Mineral | A high-quality, high-dose supplement | NeuroVite Plus |
| Omega-3 fatty acids | 1.4 grams (or more) a day of a combination of EPA and DHA in about a 60/40 ratio | Omega-3 Power<br>Omega-3 Power Squeeze |
| A combination of:<br>Ginkgo biloba<br>Acetyl-l-carnitine<br>Huperzine A<br>N-acetyl-cysteine<br>Alpha lipoic acid<br>Phosphatidylserine | | Brain and Memory Power Boost |

## EAT MORE OF THESE FOODS AND SPICES TO HEAL FROM HEAD TRAUMA

**Spices and herbs to support brain healing,** particularly turmeric, and peppermint

**Choline-rich foods to boost acetylcholine,** such as shrimp, eggs, scallops, sardines, chicken, turkey, tuna, cod, beef, collard greens, and brussels sprouts

**Omega-3-rich foods to support nerve cell membranes:** flaxseeds, walnuts, salmon, sardines, beef, shrimp, walnut oil, chia seeds, and avocado oil

**Anti-inflammatory foods:** such as **prebiotic foods** (dandelion greens, asparagus, chia seeds, beans, cabbage, psyllium, artichokes, raw garlic, onions, leeks, root vegetables—sweet potatoes, yams, squash, jicama, beets, carrots, turnips) and **probiotic-rich foods** (brined vegetables—not vinegar), kimchi, sauerkraut, kefir, miso soup, pickles, spirulina, chlorella, blue-green algae, kombucha tea)

**Zinc-rich foods:** oysters, beef, lamb, spinach, shiitake and cremini mushrooms, asparagus, sesame, and pumpkin seeds

# DAY 17. BRIGHT MINDS STRATEGY: DETOXIFY YOUR BRAIN AND BODY

Your brain is the most metabolically active organ in your body. As such, it can be damaged from environmental toxins. Exposure to environmental toxins increases the risk of psychiatric symptoms, memory problems, and dementia. Limiting or eliminating your exposure to toxins is critical to your well-being.

**YOUR PERSONAL RISK CHECKLIST**
**Which Toxins Have You Been Exposed To?**

*Place a checkmark next to any of the following toxins you have been exposed to.*

Toxins can be inhaled, absorbed through the skin, or ingested (when you eat or drink). You may have been exposed to a toxin once, on occasion, or on an ongoing basis. Below is a partial list of common toxins. Check all of the toxins that you have been exposed to so you will have a better understanding of your risk of toxic exposure.

- ☐ Air pollution
- ☐ Asbestos
- ☐ Automobile exhaust
- ☐ Aviation fumes
- ☐ Carbon monoxide
- ☐ Cigarette smoke, secondhand smoke, marijuana smoke
- ☐ Cleaning chemicals
- ☐ Fire retardant fumes
- ☐ Fire and smoke toxins (often inhaled by firefighters)
- ☐ Gasoline fumes
- ☐ Mold
- ☐ Paint and solvent fumes
- ☐ Welding or soldering fumes
- ☐ Pesticides
- ☐ Herbicides
- ☐ Pesticide or herbicide residues (farms, backyards)
- ☐ Artificial food dyes, preservatives, and sweeteners
- ☐ Foods manufactured with plastic equipment, leaking plasticizers
- ☐ BPAs (or bisphenol-A; found in plastics, food and drink containers, dental sealants, and the coating of cash register receipts)
- ☐ Chemotherapy
- ☐ General anesthesia
- ☐ Heavy metals (such as lead, mercury from dental fillings, cadmium)

- ☐ Excessive alcohol
- ☐ Many health and beauty products (such as lead in lip products, formaldehyde in nail polishes)
- ☐ Many medications (such as benzodiazepines for anxiety or insomnia, narcotics for pain)
- ☐ Marijuana
- ☐ MSG (monosodium glutamate)
- ☐ PCBs
- ☐ Polluted or tainted water (including lead and arsenic)
- ☐ Silicone breast implants that leaked

**KEY TOXIN TESTS**

The organs that detoxify your body—especially the liver, kidneys, and skin—need to be supported to do their job. The tests below will tell you how these organs are coping with your body's toxic load.

### Liver Function
- ☐ ALT (SGPT): Normal range: 7 - 56 units per liter (U/L)
- ☐ AST (SGOT): Normal range: 5 - 40 U/L
- ☐ Bilirubin: Normal range: 0.2 - 1.2 mg/dL
- ☐ Zinc: Normal range: 60 - 110 mcg/dL (low zinc will limit detoxification in the liver)

### Kidney Function
- ☐ BUN: Normal range: 7 - 20 mg/dL
- ☐ Creatinine: Normal range: 0.5 - 1.2 mg/dL

### Skin
- ☐ Check for rashes, acne, and rosacea—clues to detoxification problems

### Testing for Mold
- ☐ TGF beta-1: Normal level: below 2,380; 0 is optimal. Mold exposure can raise this to more than 15,000
- ☐ Real Time Labs mycotoxin test (http://www.realtimelab.com/ home): for mold tests of human and environmental samples

### Testing for Heavy Metals
- ☐ Hair sample and urinary "challenge" tests are common

**STRATEGIES TO REDUCE YOUR TOXINS RISK**
*Day 17 Exercise: Choose at least 1 of the following strategies to start today.*

- ☐ Quit smoking
- ☐ Address drug and alcohol abuse
- ☐ Limit alcohol to no more than 2-4 normal size drinks a week
- ☐ Remove amalgam dental fillings
- ☐ Avoid aluminum and Teflon cookware
- ☐ Buy and store foods in glass jars when possible
- ☐ Go organic
- ☐ Avoid foods with chemicals, additives, and preservatives
- ☐ Avoid processed meats
- ☐ Do a food detox
- ☐ Use an air purifier
- ☐ Eliminate unsafe health, beauty, and personal care products
- ☐ Check for mold in your home
- ☐ Use the Environmental Working Group's Skin Deep database (ewg.org/skindeep)
- ☐ Use the Think Dirty app (thinkdirtyapp.com)
- ☐ Support your liver: Limit alcohol and eat brassicas (Brussels sprouts, cabbage, broccoli, cauliflower)
- ☐ Support your kidneys: Drink 3-4 quarts of clean water a day
- ☐ Support your skin: Work up a sweat when you exercise or take a sauna

**NUTRACEUTICALS TO SUPPORT BRAIN HEALING**

**GUT (See Day 14)**

**LIVER**

| SUPPLEMENT | RECOMMENDED DOSAGE | BRAINMD SOLUTIONS |
|---|---|---|
| N-acetyl-cysteine | 600 mg twice a day | Brain and Memory Power Boost |
| Vitamin C | 1,000 mg twice a day | NeuroC, NeuroVite Plus |

**KIDNEYS**

| SUPPLEMENT | RECOMMENDED DOSAGE | BRAINMD SOLUTIONS |
|---|---|---|
| Magnesium glycinate, citrate, or malate | 200 mg twice a day | Magnesium Chewables |
| Ginkgo biloba extract | 60 mg twice a day | Brain and Memory Power Boost |

**SKIN**

| SUPPLEMENT | RECOMMENDED DOSAGE | BRAINMD SOLUTIONS |
|---|---|---|
| Vitamin D | 2,000 IU a day or more, depending on your level | Vitamin D3 |
| Vitamin E | 60 mg of mixed tocopherols a day | NeuroVite Plus |
| Omega-3 fatty acids | 1.4 grams (or more) a day combination of EPA, DHA in about a 60/40 ratio | Omega-3 Power, Omega-3 Power Squeeze |

## EAT MORE—OR LESS—OF THESE FOODS AND SPICES TO SUPPORT DETOXIFICATION
*Day 17 Exercise: Check which of the following foods you will add to your diet.*

### FOR A HEALTHIER LIVER
**Eat More:**
- ☐ Green leafy vegetables (for folate)
- ☐ Protein-rich foods, including eggs
- ☐ Brassicas: any color cabbage, brussels sprouts, cauliflower, broccoli, kale for detox
- ☐ Oranges and tangerines
- ☐ Berries
- ☐ Sunflower and sesame seeds
- ☐ Caraway and dill seeds

**Eat Less:**
- ☐ Processed meats
- ☐ Grapefruit
- ☐ Capsaicin (from red chili peppers)
- ☐ Conventionally raised produce
- ☐ Dairy
- ☐ Grain-fed meats
- ☐ Farmed fish

### FOR HEALTHIER KIDNEYS
**Eat More:**
- ☐ Water
- ☐ Spices to support detoxification: clove, rosemary, turmeric
- ☐ Nuts and seeds: cashews, almonds, and pumpkin seeds for magnesium
- ☐ Green leafy vegetables
- ☐ Citrus fruits, except grapefruit
- ☐ Beet juice
- ☐ Ginger
- ☐ Blueberries, raspberries, strawberries, blackberries
- ☐ Garlic
- ☐ Sugar-free chocolate

# DAY 18: BRIGHT MINDS STRATEGY: STABILIZE YOUR MOODS – MIND-STORMS

Your brain is the world's most powerful hybrid electrochemical engine. It uses electricity and neurotransmitters to help you think, feel, and act. Some diseases of the brain start by damaging the brain's wiring or impairing the ability to create the right amount of electricity.

**YOUR PERSONAL CHECKLIST**
**Which mind-storms risk factors do you have?**

*Place a checkmark next to any of the following issues you have or have had in the past.*

- ☐ Seizures or history of seizures
- ☐ Periods of spaciness or confusion
- ☐ Frequent complaints that things look, sound, taste, smell, or feel "funny"
- ☐ Sudden, repeated fear or anger
- ☐ Irritability that tends to build, explode, then recede, often leaving one feeling tired after a rage
- ☐ Periods of panic and/or fear for no specific reason
- ☐ Visual or auditory changes, such as seeing shadows or hearing muffled sounds
- ☐ Frequent periods of déjà vu (feelings of being somewhere you have never been)
- ☐ Mild paranoia
- ☐ Headaches or abdominal pain of uncertain origin

**KEY MIND-STORMS TESTS.**

- ☐ Brain imaging
- ☐ Irlen syndrome

**STRATEGIES THAT DECREASE MIND-STORMS**
*Day 18 Exercise: Choose at least 1 of the following strategies to start today.*

- ☐ **Ketogenic diet:** The main idea of a "keto" diet is for you to get more calories from protein and fat and significantly less from carbohydrates. When you eat less than 50 grams of carbohydrates a day, your body runs out of blood sugars and eventually (usually after 3-4 days) starts to break down protein and fat for energy. This is called ketosis. People use this diet most often to lose weight because it takes more calories to convert fat into energy than carbohydrates and helps you feel fuller longer, but it has also been shown to help seizures.
- ☐ **Neurofeedback:** This non-invasive treatment may help calm electrical activity in the brain by training you to gain control of your brain waves through self-regulation.

- ☐ **Avoid anything that increases the risk of mind-storms:**
- ☐ Excessive stress
- ☐ Lack of sleep
- ☐ Forgetting medications
- ☐ Hyperventilating
- ☐ Alcohol and drug abuse
- ☐ Dietary sugar
- ☐ Low or high blood sugar states
- ☐ Missing meals
- ☐ Red dye, monosodium glutamate (MSG)
- ☐ Premenstrual syndrome
- ☐ Illnesses
- ☐ Pain
- ☐ Video games for vulnerable brains
- ☐ Excessive screen time

**NUTRACEUTICALS TO SUPPORT BRAIN HEALING**

| SUPPLEMENT | RECOMMENDED DOSAGE | BRAINMD SOLUTIONS |
|---|---|---|
| Magnesium | 50-400 mg a day | Magnesium Chewables |
| GABA | 100-1,500 mg a day for adults; 50-750 mg a day for children | GABA Calming Support |

# DAY 19: BRIGHT MINDS STRATEGY: BOOST IMMUNITY TO PROTECT AGAINST INFECTIONS

This risk factor is all about your body's defender, the immune system, which is always on the lookout for external invaders and internal troublemakers. When your immunity isn't what it should be, you may be more vulnerable to allergies, autoimmune disorders, and infections, and the last 2 can increase your risk of brain health and mental health problems, including:

- Anxiety
- Depression
- ADD/ADHD
- Bipolar disorder
- OCD
- Tourette's syndrome
- Dementia, including Alzheimer's
- Schizophrenia
- Suicidal thoughts

**YOUR PERSONAL CHECKLIST**
**Which Immunity and Infection Risk Factors Do You Have?**

*Place a checkmark next to any of the following conditions you have or have had in the past.*

- ☐ Autoimmune disorders, such as:
    - o Multiple sclerosis
    - o Rheumatoid arthritis
    - o Systemic lupus erythematosus
    - o Crohn's disease
    - o Psoriasis
    - o Hashimoto's thyroiditis
    - o Type 1 diabetes

- ☐ Unidentified infections, such as:
    - o Lyme disease
    - o Toxoplasmosis
    - o Candida (fungal) infections
    - o Syphilis
    - o PANDAS (or PANS)
    - o Helicobacter pylori (H. pylori)
    - o HIV/AIDS
    - o Herpes

- ☐ Low vitamin D level
- ☐ Asthma and hay fever
- ☐ Allergies to gluten, peanuts, corn, soy, and other foods and substances

**KEY TESTS OF IMMUNITY/INFECTIOUS DISEASE**
- ☐ Complete blood count with differential
- ☐ Erythrocyte sedimentation rate (ESR)
- ☐ Antinuclear antibodies (ANA)
- ☐ Vitamin D: A normal level is 30-100 ng/mL; optimal level is 50-100 ng/mL

**Get tested for common infections:** If your mind (or a loved one's mind) isn't getting better with standard treatment and you don't have the benefit of a SPECT scan, consider getting screened for infectious diseases that commonly affect the mind, such as:

- ☐ Borrelia burgdorferi (the spirochete that causes Lyme disease)
- ☐ HIV/AIDS
- ☐ Syphilis
- ☐ Herpes simplex 1 and 2
- ☐ Cytomegalovirus
- ☐ Epstein-Barr virus
- ☐ Toxoplasma gondii
- ☐ H. pylori
- ☐ Chlamydophila pneumoniae
- ☐ Candidiasis

**STRATEGIES TO STRENGTHEN THE IMMUNE SYSTEM**
*Day 19 Exercise: Choose at least 1 of the following strategies to start today.*

- ☐ Work with an integrative or functional medicine doctor to properly diagnose and treat you
- ☐ Try an elimination diet (see below)
- ☐ Consider getting tested for heavy metals
- ☐ Address any gut issues you may have
- ☐ Make sure your vitamin D levels are optimal
- ☐ Manage your stress with laughter, among other strategies

## NUTRACEUTICALS TO SUPPORT BRAIN HEALING

| SUPPLEMENT | RECOMMENDED DOSAGE | BRAINMD SOLUTIONS |
|---|---|---|
| Therapeutic mushrooms (such as lion's mane, shiitake, reishi, and cordyceps) | | Smart Mushrooms |
| Probiotics | 1.4 grams (or more) a day of a combination of EPA and DHA in about a 60/40 ratio | ProBrainBiotics |
| Vitamins C, D, and E | | NeuroVite Plus, Vitamin D |
| Zinc | | NeuroVite Plus |

## EAT MORE OF THESE IMMUNITY-BOOSTING FOODS AND SPICES

**Immunity-boosting spices:** cinnamon, garlic, turmeric, thyme, ginger, coriander
**Allicin-rich foods:** raw, crushed garlic, onions, and shallots
**Quercetin-rich foods:** red onions, red cabbage, red apples, cherries, red grapes, cherry tomatoes, teas, lemons, celery, and cocoa
**Vitamin C–rich foods:** natural blood thinners to boost circulation, including oranges, tangerines, kiwifruit, berries, red and yellow bell peppers, dark green leafy vegetables (such as spinach and kale), broccoli, tomatoes, peas
**Vitamin D–rich foods:** fatty fish, including salmon, sardines, tuna, eggs, beef liver, cod liver oil
**Zinc-rich foods:** oysters, beef, lamb, spinach, shiitake and cremini mushrooms, asparagus, sesame, and pumpkin seeds
**Mushrooms:** shiitake, white button, portabella, morel, chanterelle
**Selenium-rich foods:** nuts (especially Brazil nuts), seeds, fish, grass-fed meats, mushrooms
**Omega 3–rich foods:** flaxseeds, walnuts, salmon, sardines, beef, shrimp, walnut oil, chia seeds, avocado oil
**Prebiotic-rich foods:** dandelion greens, asparagus, chia seeds, beans, cabbage, psyllium, artichokes, raw garlic, onions, leeks, root vegetables (sweet potatoes, yams, squash, jicama, beets, carrots, turnips)
**Probiotic-rich foods:** (brined vegetables—not vinegar), kimchi, sauerkraut, kefir, miso soup, pickles, spirulina, chlorella, blue-green algae, kombucha tea)

*Day 19 Exercise: Try an elimination diet for 1 month.*
**STRATEGIES THAT DECREASE MIND-STORMS**

1. Cut out the 6 potential food allergens (sugar, artificial sweeteners, gluten, soy, corn, milk) for one month.

2. After a month, slowly reintroduce food items one at a time every 3-4 days. Eat the reintroduced food at least 2-3 times a day for 3 days to see if you notice a reaction.

3. Look for symptoms, which can occur within a few minutes up to 72 hours later. (If you notice a problem right away, stop consuming that food immediately.) Reactions to foods to which you have allergies can include:
- ☐ brain fog
- ☐ difficulty remembering
- ☐ mood issues (anxiety, depression, and anger)
- ☐ nasal congestion
- ☐ chest congestion
- ☐ headaches
- ☐ sleep problems
- ☐ joint aches
- ☐ muscle aches
- ☐ pain
- ☐ fatigue
- ☐ skin changes
- ☐ changes in digestion and bowel functioning

4. If you have a reaction, note the food and eliminate it for 90 days, and maybe forever. This will give your immune system a chance to cool off and your gut a chance to heal.

# DAY 20. BRIGHT MINDS STRATEGY: OPTIMIZE YOUR NEUROHORMONES

Hormones are messengers—chemicals that are made by different parts of the body and sent to other areas to control your body's basic functions. The brain plays a significant role, both in sending out signals to release hormones and in being influenced by hormones from other areas of the body. Hormones work together in a delicate balance that can be upset if too much or too little of one or more is produced. You may experience symptoms that affect how you feel, think, or act, and you may be more prone to depression, Alzheimer's disease, diabetes, and other illnesses.

When hormones are balanced, it helps you feel balanced. When hormones are out of balance, you may experience symptoms related to:

- Anxiety
- Depression
- Low motivation
- Lack of focus
- Memory problems
- Brain fog

**YOUR PERSONAL CHECKLIST:**
**Which Neurohormone Risk Factors Do You Have?**
There are literally hundreds of hormones that influence your brain, but these six are the most important: thyroid, cortisol/DHEA, estrogen, progesterone, and testosterone. Here are some of the risk factors you could have (you may not know you have one or more of them without laboratory testing):

- ☐ Underactive thyroid
- ☐ Overactive thyroid
- ☐ Elevated cortisol and low DHEA (adrenal fatigue)
- ☐ Low estrogen
- ☐ Excess estrogen
- ☐ Low progesterone
- ☐ Perimenopause
- ☐ Menopause
- ☐ Low testosterone
- ☐ Excess testosterone

**KEY NEUROHORMONE TESTS**
- ☐ Thyroid panel (includes TSH, Free T3, Free T4, and Thyroid antibodies)
- ☐ Liver function tests
- ☐ Ferritin level
- ☐ Cortisol
- ☐ DHEA-S (note that normal blood levels can differ by age and sex)
- ☐ Free and total serum testosterone (men and women)
- ☐ Estrogen and progesterone (women only)

**STRATEGIES TO KEEP NEUROHORMONES HEALTHY**
*Day 20 Exercise: Choose at least 1 of the following strategies to start today*

- ☐ Limit or eliminate:
  - o Smoking (which lowers the age of menopause)
  - o Chronic stress
  - o Processed food
  - o Too much sugar
  - o Unhealthy fats
  - o Wheat
  - o Obesity
  - o Caffeine
  - o Alcohol
  - o Endocrine disruptors (pesticides, plastics, fragrances in health and beauty products, etc.)
- ☐ Exercise aerobically and lift weights
- ☐ Get 7-8 hours of sleep every night
- ☐ Try to manage your stress
- ☐ Eat a healthy diet
- ☐ Buy organic food
- ☐ Check the Environmental Working Group (www.ewg.org) for fruits and vegetables with the highest and lowest pesticide levels
- ☐ Avoid buying and storing food in plastic containers
- ☐ Limit or avoid conventionally raised produce and dairy
- ☐ When taking hormone supplements, opt for bio-identical ones (they have fewer side effects)

**NUTRACEUTICALS TO SUPPORT BRAIN HEALING**

| SUPPLEMENT | RECOMMENDED DOSAGE | BRAINMD SOLUTIONS |
|---|---|---|
| L-tyrosine | 500-1,000 mg a day | Tyrosine |
| Zinc | 25 mg a day | NeuroVite Plus |
| DHEA | 25-50 mg a day (as determined by lab testing) | |

**EAT MORE OF THESE NEUROHORMONE-BALANCING FOODS AND SPICES**

**Fiber-rich foods, including those that contain lignin:** green beans, peas, carrots, seeds, Brazil nuts

**Hormone-supporting spices:** garlic, sage, parsley, anise seed, red clover, hops, eggs

**Testosterone-boosting foods:** pomegranates, olive oil, oysters, coconut, brassicas (including cabbage, broccoli, brussels sprouts, cauliflower), whey protein, garlic

**Estrogen-boosting foods:** soybeans, flaxseeds, sunflower seeds, beans, garlic, yams, foods rich in vitamins C and Bs, beets, parsley, aniseed, red clover, hops, sage

**Thyroid-boosting (selenium-rich) foods:** seaweed and sea vegetables, brassicas, maca

**Progesterone-boosting foods:** chasteberry, plus magnesium-rich foods

**Zinc-rich foods to boost testosterone:** oysters, beef, lamb, spinach, shiitake and cremini mushrooms, asparagus, sesame and pumpkin seeds

**Prebiotic-rich foods:** dandelion greens, asparagus, chia seeds, beans, cabbage, psyllium, artichokes, raw garlic, onions, leeks, root vegetables (sweet potatoes, yams, squash, jicama, beets, carrots, turnips), and probiotic-rich foods

**Probiotic-rich foods:** (brined vegetables—not vinegar), kimchi, sauerkraut, kefir, miso soup, pickles, spirulina, chlorella, blue-green algae, kombucha tea)

# DAY 21. BRIGHT MINDS STRATEGY: ACHIEVE HEALTHY WEIGHT AND BLOOD SUGAR TO PREVENT DIABESITY

The word "diabesity" combine diabetes and obesity, both of which negatively impact brain health. Amen Clinics research using brain imaging shows that as weight goes up, the physical size and function of the brain goes down. Diabetes and obesity are associated with a greater risk of mental and cognitive health issues.

Diabesity is linked to an increased risk of:

- Anxiety
- Depression
- Bipolar disorder
- Addictions
- Alzheimer's disease and other dementias

**YOUR PERSONAL CHECKLIST:**
**Which Diabesity Risk Factors Do You Have?**
*Place a checkmark next to your risk factors.*

- ☐ Aging
- ☐ Family history of diabetes
- ☐ Excessive consumption of sugar and high-glycemic foods
- ☐ Obesity
- ☐ Alcohol abuse
- ☐ Exposure to toxins
- ☐ Sedentary lifestyle
- ☐ Metabolic syndrome

**KEY DIABESITY TESTS**

- ☐ Body mass index (BMI) (see Day 5)
- ☐ Waist to height ratio (see Day 5)
- ☐ Hemoglobin A1C (HbA1C) (see Day 5)
- ☐ Vitamin D level (see Day 5)
- ☐ Fasting blood sugar
- ☐ Normal: 70-105 mg/dL
- ☐ Optimal: 70-89 mg/dL
- ☐ Prediabetes: 105-125 mg/dL
- ☐ Diabetes: 126 mg/dL or higher

- ☐ Fasting Insulin
- ☐ Normal: 2.6-25
- ☐ Optimal: Less than 10

## STRATEGIES TO COMBAT DIABESITY
*Day 21 Exercise: Choose at least 1 of the following strategies to start today.*

- ☐ Follow a brain healthy diet
- ☐ Limit low-fiber foods, sugar and foods that turn to sugar, wheat and other grains, and processed foods
- ☐ If you're overweight, lose weight slowly (1-2 pounds a week)
- ☐ Drink more water—and don't drink your calories
- ☐ Take saunas to help detoxify
- ☐ Exercise aerobically and do strength training
- ☐ See your doctor to find out if medication is necessary
- ☐ On BrainFitLife, use hypnosis before bedtime to calm your mind
- ☐ Avoid the diabesity mind-set (see exercise below)

## NUTRACEUTICALS TO SUPPORT BRAIN HEALING

| SUPPLEMENT | RECOMMENDED DOSAGE | BRAINMD SOLUTIONS |
|---|---|---|
| Omega-3 fatty acids | 1.4 grams (or more) a day of a combination of EPA and DHA in about a 60/40 ratio | Omega-3 Power<br>Omega-3 Power Squeeze |
| Chromium picolinate | 200-1,000 mcg a day | Craving Control<br>NeuroVite Plus<br>Brain & Body Power Max |
| Cinnamon | 1-6 g a day | |

## EAT MORE OF THESE NEUROHORMONE-BALANCING FOODS AND SPICES

**Spices:** cinnamon, turmeric, ginger, cumin, garlic, cayenne, oregano, marjoram, sage, nutmeg

**Fiber-rich foods to balance cholesterol and blood pressure:** psyllium husk, navy beans, raspberries, broccoli, spinach, lentils, green peas, pears, winter squash, cabbage, green beans, avocados, coconut, fresh figs, artichokes, chickpeas, hemp seeds, and chia seeds

**Polyphenol-rich foods/drinks,** especially green tea, decaffeinated coffee, and blueberries.

**Protein-rich foods:** eggs, meats, fish

**Vegetables: Best choices:** celery, spinach, and brassicas (broccoli, Brussels sprouts, cauliflower)

**Fruits:** apples, oranges, blueberries, raspberries, blackberries, and strawberries

**Omega-3-rich foods:** flaxseeds, walnuts, salmon, sardines, beef, shrimp, walnut oil, chia seeds, avocado oil

**Magnesium-rich foods:** pumpkin and sunflower seeds, almonds, spinach, Swiss chard, sesame seeds, beet greens, summer squash, quinoa, black beans, and cashews

**Vitamin D-rich foods:** fatty fish, including salmon, sardines, tuna; eggs; mushrooms (maitake, morel, shiitake); beef liver, cod liver oil

***Day 21 Exercise: Avoid the mindset of diabesity. In the chart below, write down your Diabesity Mindset thoughts and how you can change those thoughts to serve you better.***

These are beliefs and thoughts you tell yourself that increase the risk you will never truly get healthy, such as:

- "Everything in moderation," which is generally the thought just before you are going to eat something that will hurt you.

- "Live a little, you deserve it." Funny, but this is the thought of early death. It should be rephrased as "Live a little shorter."

- "I want what I want when I want it" is a 4-year-old's mindset, but this thought underlies why most people do not get healthy. We need to be good parents to ourselves and be firm about engaging in good behavior if we want to end mental illness.

- "But I always do it this way," is another common thought that tells you that your habits are destroying your mind.

EXAMPLE:

| DIABESITY MINDSET | HEALTHY MINDSET |
|---|---|
| "I just want to have fun." | Who really has more fun? The person with the troubled brain or the one with the healthy brain? No question, it's the one with the healthy brain! |

| DIABESITY MINDSET | HEALTHY MINDSET |
|---|---|
|  |  |

# Week 4

# DAY 22: BRIGHT MINDS STRATEGY: SLEEP

Sleep plays a critical role in your moods, emotions, stress levels, and your ability to control your dragons. A lack of sleep can fuel your dragons and make you feel sad, irritable, anxious, overwhelmed, and stressed. It can also make it hard to concentrate and can prolong grief.

Getting the sleep you need requires 3 strategies:

1. Sleep envy (you have to see it as critically important)
2. Avoid sleep robbers
3. Engage in sleep enhancers

**YOUR PERSONAL CHECKLIST**
**Which Sleep Risk Factors Do You Have?**
*Place a checkmark next to the risk factors you have.*

- ☐ Insomnia
- ☐ Sleep apnea
- ☐ Poor sleep hygiene
- ☐ Shift work
- ☐ Depression
- ☐ Hormonal imbalances

**KEY SLEEP TESTS**

- ☐ Get evaluated for sleep apnea (If you snore loudly, stop breathing at night, or are chronically tired in the daytime)
- ☐ Assess the number of hours of sleep you need

**STRATEGIES TO PROMOTE HEALTHY SLEEP**
**1. Avoid Sleep Robbers**
***Day 22 Exercise: Choose at least 1 of the following sleep robbers to eliminate today.***

In our hectic, 24/7 society, we could just as easily ask, "What doesn't cause sleep deprivation?" There are seemingly an endless number of reasons why millions of us are missing out on a good night's sleep. Here is a list of some of the most common factors.

- ☐ A warm room.
- ☐ Light in the bedroom.
- ☐ Noise.
- ☐ Gadgets by the bed.

- ☐ Going to bed worried or angry.
- ☐ Medications: Many medications including asthma medications, antihistamines, cough medicines, anticonvulsants, stimulants (such as Adderall or Concerta prescribed for ADHD), and many others disturb sleep.
- ☐ Caffeine: Too much caffeine from coffee, tea, chocolate, or some herbal preparations — especially when consumed later in the day or at night — can disrupt sleep.
- ☐ Alcohol, nicotine, and marijuana: Although these compounds initially induce sleepiness for some people, they have the reverse effect as they wear off, which is why you may wake up several hours after you go to sleep.
- ☐ Restless Legs Syndrome: A nighttime jerking or pedaling motion of the legs that drives a person's bed partner crazy (as well as the person who has it).
- ☐ Women's issues: Pregnancy, PMS, menopause, and perimenopause cause fluctuations in hormone levels that can disrupt the sleep cycle.
- ☐ Thyroid conditions.
- ☐ Congestive heart failure.
- ☐ Chronic pain conditions.
- ☐ Untreated or undertreated psychiatric conditions such as obsessive-compulsive disorder, depression, or anxiety.
- ☐ Alzheimer's disease: Dementia patients "sundown" or rev up at night and wander.
- ☐ Chronic gastrointestinal problems, such as reflux.
- ☐ Men's issues: Benign prostatic hypertrophy causes many trips to the bathroom at night, which interrupts slumber.
- ☐ Snoring: It can wake you or your sleep mate, or everyone in the house if it is really loud.
- ☐ Sleep apnea: With this condition, you stop breathing for short periods of time throughout the night, which robs you of restful sleep and leaves you feeling sluggish, inattentive, and forgetful throughout the day.
- ☐ Shift work: Nurses, firefighters, security personnel, customer service representatives, truck drivers, airline pilots, and many others toil by night and sleep by day. Or, at least, they try to sleep. Shift workers are especially vulnerable to irregular sleep patterns, which leads to excessive sleepiness, reduced productivity, irritability, and mood problems.
- ☐ Stressful events: The death of a loved one, divorce, a major deadline at work, or an upcoming test can cause temporary sleep loss.
- ☐ Jet lag: International travel across time zones wreaks havoc with sleep cycles.

## 2. Engage in Sleep Enhancers
*Day 22 Exercise: Choose at least 1 of the following sleep enhancers to start today.*

Here are 21 ways to make it easier to drift off to dreamland and get a good night's sleep. Remember that we are all unique individuals and what works for one person may not work for another. Keep trying new techniques until you find something that works.

- ☐ A cooler room.
- ☐ A completely dark bedroom.
- ☐ Make the room noise free or wear ear plugs.
- ☐ Turn off the gadgets by the bed, or at least turn off the sound.
- ☐ Try to fix emotional problems before going to sleep with a positive text, email, or intention to deal with the issue tomorrow. If you forgive the other person first, you may just end the argument.
- ☐ Maintain a regular sleep schedule — going to bed at the same time each night and waking up at the same time each day, including on weekends. Get up at the same time each day regardless of sleep duration the previous night.
- ☐ Create a soothing nighttime routine that encourages sleep. A warm bath, meditation, or massage can help you relax.
- ☐ Some people like to read themselves to sleep. If you are reading, make sure it isn't an action-packed thriller or a horror story — they aren't likely to help you drift off to sleep.
- ☐ If you are having trouble sleeping, don't take naps! This is one of the biggest mistakes you can make if you have insomnia. Taking naps when you feel sleepy during the day compounds the nighttime sleep cycle disruption.
- ☐ Sound therapy can induce a very peaceful mood and lull you to sleep. Consider soothing nature sounds, wind chimes, a fan, or soft music. Studies have shown that slower classical music, or any music that has a slow rhythm of 60 to 80 beats per minute, can help with sleep. You can find sleep enhancing music by Grammy award winning producer Barry Goldstein on Brain Fit Life (mybrainfitlife.com).
- ☐ Drink a mixture of warm unsweetened almond milk, a teaspoon of vanilla (the real stuff, not imitation), and a few drops of stevia. This may increase serotonin in your brain and help you sleep.
- ☐ Don't eat for at least 2-3 hours before going to bed.
- ☐ Regular exercise is very beneficial for insomnia, but don't do it within four hours of the time you hit the sack. Vigorous exercise late in the evening may energize you and keep you awake.
- ☐ Take a warm bath or shower before bed.
- ☐ Wear socks to bed. Researchers have found that warm hands and feet were the best predictor of rapid sleep onset.
- ☐ Don't drink any caffeinated beverages in the afternoon or evening. Also avoid chocolate, nicotine, and alcohol—especially at night. Although alcohol can initially make you feel sleepy, it actually interrupts sleep.

- ☐ If you wake up in the middle of the night, refrain from looking at the clock. Checking the time can make you feel anxious, which aggravates the problem.
- ☐ Use the bed and bedroom only for sleep or sexual activity. Sexual activity releases many natural hormones, releases muscle tension, and boosts a sense of well-being. Adults with healthy sex lives tend to sleep better. When you are unable to fall asleep or return to sleep easily, get up and go to another room.
- ☐ Hypnosis or meditation can help. We have audio downloads on Brain Fit Life (mybrainfitlife.com) that could be helpful.
- ☐ Use the scent of lavender to enhance sleep. It has been shown to decrease anxiety and improve mood and sleep.
- ☐ If you have to resort to medication, stay away from the benzodiazepines and traditional sleep medications. I often use propranolol, Remeron, and trazodone.

**NUTRACEUTICALS TO PROMOTE HEALTHY SLEEP**

| SUPPLEMENT | RECOMMENDED DOSAGE | BRAINMD SOLUTIONS |
|---|---|---|
| Melatonin | 0.3-6 mg (less is often better) | Put Me to Sleep<br>Restful Sleep |
| 5-HTP (especially for worriers) | 50-200 mg | Put Me to Sleep<br>Restful Sleep |
| Magnesium glycinate or citrate | 50-400 mg | Put Me to Sleep<br>Restful Sleep |
| GABA | 250-1,000 mg | Put Me to Sleep<br>Restful Sleep |

# TAME YOUR DRAGONS

Over the following 13 days, you'll learn more about your dragons, including their origins, triggers, and reactions, as well as proven strategies to tame your dragons and helpful affirmations to calm them.

# DAY 23. FINDING SIGNIFICANCE: TAMING THE ABANDONED, INVISIBLE, OR INSIGNIFICANT DRAGONS

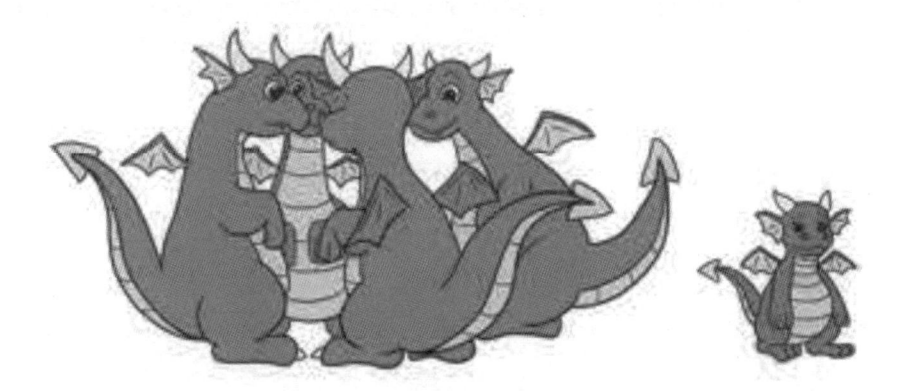

Others did not see or recognize you, or you felt unimportant, abandoned, and lonely.

| COMMON WHEN... | TRIGGERS | REACTIONS | STRATEGIES | AFFIRMATIONS |
|---|---|---|---|---|
| Your parents were unable or unavailable to raise you.<br><br>You were a middle child from a large family.<br><br>Your parents or siblings were dysfunctional, narcissistic (all about them), or sick.<br><br>One of your parents or siblings was a high achiever or famous. | When you perceive that others ignore or belittle you<br><br>When others are recognized and you are not<br><br>When you get laid off from work but your colleagues don't | Feelings of loneliness<br><br>Feelings of worthlessness<br><br>Feeling small | Know your life's purpose.<br><br>Work toward making a difference in the lives of others.<br><br>Become part of a group (church, civic, etc.).<br><br>Psychotherapy | I am loved.<br><br>I am unique.<br><br>I am significant.<br><br>I am seen by... (name the people who see you).<br><br>I am making a difference in the lives of... (name them). |

If this is one of your dragons, you need to find ways to feel significant, like your life matters. Finding your purpose in life is one of the most powerful ways to do that (see Day 38 to learn how to find your purpose). Making a difference in the lives of others is another important strategy that will help you feel more significant, happy, and connected.

My Abandoned, Invisible, or Insignificant Dragons drove me to want to be connected, seen, and significant. I've worked hard over the course of my life to make a difference in others, and I love sharing what I have learned in front of large crowds. One of my favorite lectures ever was at the American Airlines Arena in front of 20,000 people. In large part, these dragons are why I wrote *Your Brain Is Always Listening* and why I created this workbook for you.

**Here are some ways to make a difference in the lives of others.**

**1. Volunteer.** Volunteering actually helps to grow the hippocampus (memory and mood) and improves a person's sense of achievement and productivity over a 2-year period. Connect meaningful activities and pleasure, such as volunteering for activities you love.
Example: I love table tennis and enjoy keeping score for others during tournaments.

**2. Become a coach or mentor.** Helping others learn from you can make you feel like your life has value. You can become a mentor in your professional field, or you can become a brain health coach by sharing what you've learned about optimizing your brain. (See the Brain Health Licensed Trainer Course at AmenUniversity.com for more information on this online course.)

*Day 23 Exercise: Write 5 ways you can make a difference in the lives of others and how it will make you feel (such as significant, seen, valued, important, or connected).*

| HOW I CAN MAKE A DIFFERENCE IN OTHER PEOPLE'S LIVES | HOW IT MAKES ME FEEL |
|---|---|
|  |  |
|  |  |
|  |  |
|  |  |
|  |  |

# DAY 24. STOP COMPARING: TAMING THE INFERIOR OR FLAWED DRAGONS

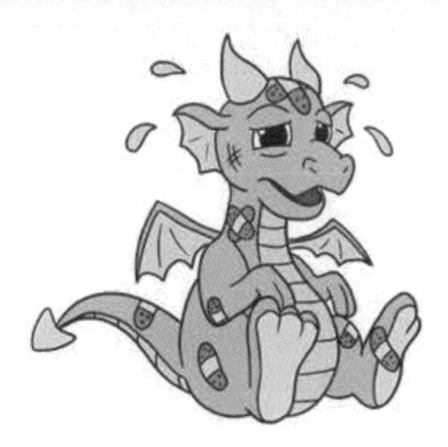

You felt "less than" others in ability, looks, money, achievement, or relationships.

| COMMON WHEN... | TRIGGERS | REACTIONS | STRATEGIES | AFFIRMATIONS |
|---|---|---|---|---|
| You felt inadequate.<br><br>You thought you could not live up to your parents' expectations.<br><br>You were bullied, cut down, or criticized by peers, family, or authority figures.<br><br>You frequently compared yourself to others in a negative way. | Comparing yourself to others<br><br>Competing against others<br><br>Looking in the mirror | Feelings of inferiority, depression, helplessness, and jealousy<br><br>Being overly sensitive or a perfectionist<br><br>Having an impostor syndrome (feeling like you're a fraud or don't know what you're doing)<br><br>Having body dysmorphic disorder, where you only see your body's flaws | Work to stop comparing yourself to others.<br><br>Stop caring what other people think of you, because they are mostly not thinking about you at all.<br><br>Realize that seeking perfection is a reason to fail. | I am unique.<br><br>I restrain comparing myself to others.<br><br>I am a strong, independent person.<br><br>I will be my best, not someone else's best.<br><br>I work hard. |

These dragons drive feelings of inferiority, depression, helplessness, and jealousy; make you overly sensitive or a perfectionist; may lead to impostor syndrome (feeling like you're a fraud or don't know what you're doing) or body dysmorphic disorder, where you see only your body's flaws.

***Day 24 Exercise: To overcome this, work to stop comparing yourself to others. Choose at least 1 of the following strategies to start today.***

- ☐ Be aware when you do it.
- ☐ Know what triggers you to compare yourself to others and avoiding them (e.g., social media, magazine/TV ads).
- ☐ Change your focus to something else.
- ☐ Focus on your strengths and accomplishments.
- ☐ Praise others because it makes it more likely you will praise yourself.
- ☐ Avoid mindlessly scrolling through social media.
- ☐ Tell yourself, "It's nobody else's job to love me. It's mine."
- ☐ Remember the 18-40-60 Rule:
    - o When you're 18, you worry about what others think of you.
    - o When you're 40, you don't care what others think of you.
    - o When you're 60, you realize nobody has been thinking of you at all, people only think of themselves.

# DAY 25. FINDING PEACE: TAMING THE ANXIOUS DRAGONS

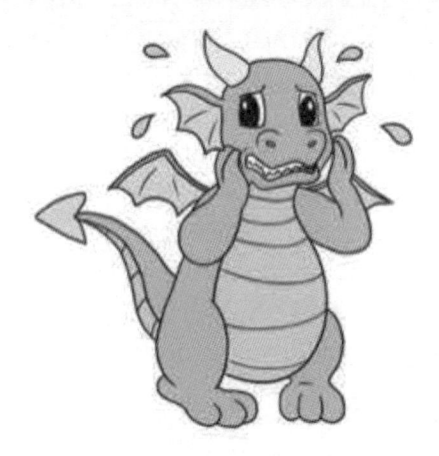

You were often afraid, had a sense of impending doom, felt overwhelmed or stressed, or thought the world was a dangerous place.

| COMMON WHEN... | TRIGGERS | REACTIONS | STRATEGIES | AFFIRMATIONS |
|---|---|---|---|---|
| You had an alcoholic or drug-addicted parent, stepparent, or sibling. You had an angry or unpredictable parent, stepparent, or sibling. You lived through the coronavirus pandemic. | Reminders of past situations that caused anxiety. Frightening events (like a global pandemic, natural disaster, or rioting in the streets) Having to speak in public Hearing loud noises Being overscheduled | Panic attacks Nervousness Phobias Predict the worst Physical symptoms (insomnia, headaches, upset stomach, cold or sweaty hands, racing heart, chest pain) Increased vulnerability to infections, illnesses Worry about being scrutinized | Diaphragmatic breathing Prayer and meditation Loving Kindness Meditation Hypnosis Use your 5 senses to calm your emotional brain | I am safe. I am secure. I am calm. I am protected. I focus on my breathing and centering myself. |

*Day 25 Exercise: Use Your 5 senses to calm your emotional brain.*

If you have Anxious Dragons, start practicing the strategies listed in the chart. (Go back to Day 9 for a refresher on how to do diaphragmatic breathing, Loving Kindness Meditation, and hypnosis.)

On this day, learn to use your senses to soothe your mind. The brain senses the world. If you can change the inputs, you can often quickly change how you feel.

- **Vision**—Look at images of nature; create a folder of images that make you feel happy.
- **Hearing**—Develop a playlist of soothing music. (See Day 9)
- **Touch**—Get a hug, massage, acupressure, or sit in a sauna for better touch inputs.
- **Smell**—Inhale calming scents, such as lavender, chamomile, rose, lemon, or jasmine. (See Day 9)
- **Tastes**—Savor chocolate, cinnamon, saffron, mint, or nutmeg.

# DAY 26. GET THE PAST OUT OF THE PRESENT: TAMING THE WOUNDED DRAGONS

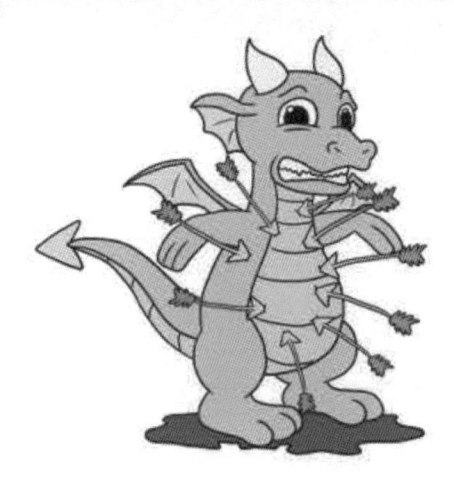

You experienced trauma or lived through intense stress.

| COMMON WHEN... | TRIGGERS | REACTIONS | STRATEGIES | AFFIRMATIONS |
|---|---|---|---|---|
| You experienced physical, emotional, or sexual abuse.<br><br>You were taken into foster care<br><br>You were in a fire, flood, or assault.<br><br>You were bullied or teased.<br><br>You lived through the coronavirus pandemic. | Anything that reminds you of the past trauma<br><br>Sights, smells, or sounds that remind you of the past trauma<br><br>Anniversaries of an accident, death, divorce, breakup, or being fired | Flashbacks and nightmares<br><br>Feeling numb<br><br>Avoiding people/places/situations that are reminders of the trauma<br><br>Watching for bad things to happen<br><br>Panic when events remotely resemble an upsetting one from the past<br><br>Inability to recall an important aspect of a past trauma<br><br>Easily startled | Know when your nervous system is out of balance and bring it back.<br><br>Try trauma-focused CBT.<br><br>Put your story on paper; tell both sides.<br><br>Stop avoiding the pain from past trauma.<br><br>Break the bonds of the past.<br><br>EMDR (Eye Movement Desensitization & Reprocessing) | I am safe in this moment.<br><br>I have everything I need in this moment.<br><br>That was then; this is now.<br><br>I release trauma, turmoil, and grief.<br><br>Asking for help is a sign of strength. |

***Day 26 Exercise: Break the bonds of the past.***

A powerful technique I use with patients who struggle with Wounded Dragons is something I call breaking the bonds of the past. It is a way to help you reframe and disconnect from past memories. Whenever your Wounded Dragons whisper painful memories inside your head, answer the following questions on a piece of paper:

When was the last time you struggled, had the painful or disruptive memory or feeling, or felt suffering? Write down the details.

_____

What were you feeling at the time? Describe the predominant feeling.

_____

When was the first time you had that feeling? In your mind, imagine yourself on a train going backward through time. Go back to the time when you first had the feeling. Write down the incident or incidents in detail.

_____

Can you go back even further to a time when you had that original feeling? Write down the details of the original incident.

_____

If you have a clear idea of the origins of the feelings, can you disconnect them by reprocessing them through an adult or parent mindset, or reframe them in light of new information? Consciously disconnect the emotional bridge to the past with the idea that what happened in the past belongs in the past, and what happens now is what matters.

_____

# DAY 27. DOES IT FIT MY GOALS? DO I WANT TO?: TAMING THE SHOULD AND SHAMING DRAGONS

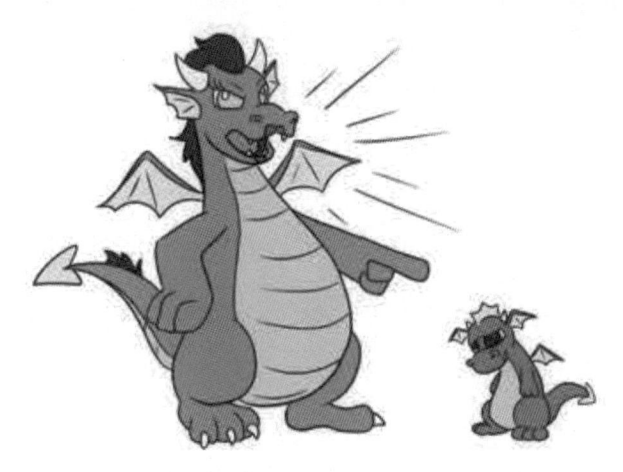

You were raised in a culture of guilt.

| COMMON WHEN... | TRIGGERS | REACTIONS | STRATEGIES | AFFIRMATIONS |
|---|---|---|---|---|
| You were humiliated, embarrassed, belittled, judged, or criticized.<br><br>You grew up in a strict religion.<br><br>You grew up in a strict culture. | Disapproval from someone important to you (parent, spouse, boss)<br><br>Perceived disapproval from God | Feeling guilty, foolish, distressed, exposed, overly sensitive, submissive<br><br>Want to hide or withdraw<br><br>Want to engage in self-harmful behaviors in secret (addictions, pornography, overeating) | Break up with the guilt.<br><br>Realize the past is the past.<br><br>Revisit your childhood.<br><br>Reflect on what triggers the feelings of shame.<br><br>Replace "should" with "I want to" or "It fits my goals to."<br><br>Talk to someone about the shame you feel.<br><br>Practice forgiveness. | Each day I feel more at peace with my past mistakes.<br><br>I work to learn the lessons of my past.<br><br>I can and will let go of any shame that haunts me.<br><br>I replace "I should do this" with "Does it fit my overall goals to do this?"<br><br>That was then, this is now. |

***Day 27 Exercise: Break up with guilt.***

Know when "should" and shame are helpful and when they are not. Do these thoughts or emotions serve you by helping you change something harmful in your life, or do they hurt you, causing you to feel like you're bad, evil, or a failure? If they do not serve you, break up with them.

Replace "should" with "I want to" or "It fits my goals to" to see if the behavior still fits. If it does, this will make you more motivated to do it. On the other hand, if an activity doesn't fit into your overall goals, you may feel more empowered by striking it from your to-do list.

Reminder: This is why the One Page Miracle (see Day 8) is so important.

*In the chart below, write down 4 of your typical "I should" statements, then replace them with "I want to" or "It fits my goals to."*

EXAMPLE:

| REPLACE "I SHOULD" | USE "I WANT TO" OR "IT FITS MY GOALS TO" |
|---|---|
| I should finish this presentation for work. | I want to finish this presentation for work because it will help me get the promotion I want. |

| REPLACE "I SHOULD" | USE "I WANT TO" OR "IT FITS MY GOALS TO" |
|---|---|
|  |  |
|  |  |
|  |  |
|  |  |

# Week 5

# DAY 28. CHANGE STARTS WITH ME: TAMING THE RESPONSIBLE DRAGONS

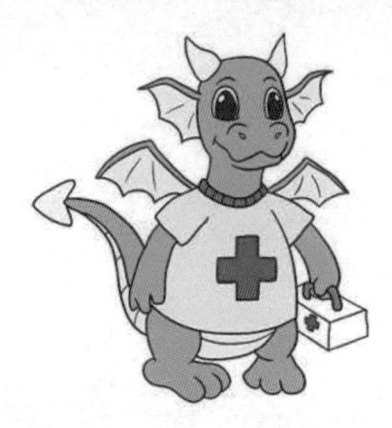

You feel liable for the pain or situation of others.

| COMMON WHEN... | TRIGGERS | REACTIONS | STRATEGIES | AFFIRMATIONS |
|---|---|---|---|---|
| You felt powerless to help someone.<br><br>You felt insignificant and fixing other's issues helped you feel significant.<br><br>If something bad happened to someone you love, you felt responsible.<br><br>You were the eldest child.<br><br>Neglectful parents made you care for siblings. | You perceive others in need | Doing too much for others<br><br>Causing others to become too dependent on you<br><br>Breeding entitlement and resentment in those you cater to<br><br>Unbalanced relationships<br><br>Long-term stress | Realize that doing too much for others can create dependency and inhibit them from being independent and self-sufficient.<br><br>Self-care is not selfish.<br><br>Evaluate the people in your life.<br><br>Deal with your past around being responsible for others. | Loving others as myself means taking care of myself so I can love others.<br><br>I love helping others, as long as I'm helping them become independent.<br><br>It is better to give than to receive, as long as giving does not create unnecessary dependency.<br><br>I share the load with others, so I don't become overburdened or burned out. |

***Day 28 Exercise: Practice self-care.***

This fixer, caretaker, codependent dragon can cause you to do too much for others, so they become dependent on you, which ultimately breeds entitlement and resentment, and creates unbalanced relationships and long-term stress.

Self-care is not selfish. Remember what they say on airplanes, "If the masks come down, put yours on first." Prioritize taking care of yourself to the same degree that you care for others. This includes setting healthy boundaries. You're limited and need to accept those limitations; otherwise, you burn out, max out, and fizzle out. If you don't, it's easy to resent those you help, seeing them as needy and taking, taking, taking all the time.

*Choose 1 of the following 25 ways to practice self-care today.*

1. Take a bath.
2. Read a book.
3. Get a massage.
4. Take a brief nap.
5. Enjoy a cup of tea.
6. Take a walk in nature.
7. Get a manicure or pedicure.
8. Try acupuncture.
9. Schedule "me" time in your planner.
10. Listen to music that relaxes you. (See Day 9)
11. Say your affirmations.
12. Knit something for yourself.
13. Go to a karate class.
14. Take a yoga class.
15. Meditate.
16. Spend time in prayer.
17. Go see a movie.
18. Take a bike ride (be sure to wear your helmet).
19. Get a haircut.
20. Get a facial.
21. Indulge your creativity—paint, write, or build something.
22. Do psychotherapy.
23. Hide out in your "man cave" or "she shed."
24. If possible, get in the water—the ocean, a lake, or a river.
25. Watch a comedy or your favorite sport.

# DAY 29. IT'S NOT ALL ABOUT YOU: TAMING THE SPECIAL, SPOILED, OR ENTITLED DRAGONS

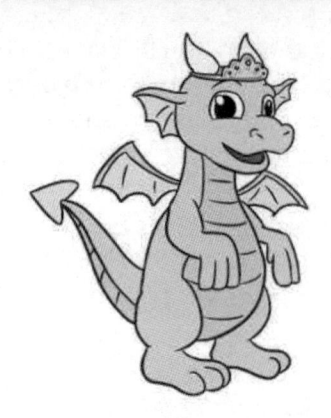

These are the "special" dragons, the golden children, favored ones, and miracle babies.

| COMMON WHEN... | TRIGGERS | REACTIONS | STRATEGIES | AFFIRMATIONS |
|---|---|---|---|---|
| Your parents wanted/loved you so much they never told you no.<br><br>You could do no wrong, and ended up with an artificially elevated sense of entitlement.<br><br>Your caregivers never wanted you to feel pain, did everything for you.<br><br>You become famous at a young age. | When you don't get your way<br><br>When others try to make you take responsibility<br><br>When you don't feel; as though you are treated as special | Lack of empathy for others<br><br>Thinking others don't matter much<br><br>Tantrums, anger, rudeness<br><br>Needing attention<br><br>A sense of injustice or outrage | Take responsibility for your life.<br><br>Change the phrase "I deserve ..." to "I am responsible ..."<br><br>Notice how good it feels to promote the success of other people.<br><br>Practice seeing things from others' point of view.<br><br>Catch yourself justifying your spoiled actions.<br><br>Spend less time around people who act entitled. | I am special, but so is everyone around me.<br><br>I am responsible for my own happiness.<br><br>I encourage the success of others.<br><br>I see things from the other person's point of view.<br><br>Acting spoiled spoils my own happiness and joy. |

**Day 29 Exercise: Take responsibility.**

You may have a lack of empathy for others, thinking others don't matter much and they are easy to cut off; tantrums, anger, rudeness, a strong need for attention, or a sense of injustice and outrage. You often say, "You owe me . . . ," "I deserve . . . ," or "It's their fault . . ."

Take responsibility for your life. Responsibility is not about fault, but rather about your ability to respond.

In the chart below, write down 5 of your typical "I deserve..." phrases and change them to "I am responsible..."

EXAMPLE:

| I DESERVE... | I AM RESPONSIBLE FOR... |
|---|---|
| I deserve a promotion. | I am responsible for doing work that helps me get a promotion. |

| I DESERVE... | I AM RESPONSIBLE FOR... |
|---|---|
|  |  |
|  |  |
|  |  |
|  |  |
|  |  |

SIX WEEKS TO OVERCOME ANXIETY, DEPRESSION, TRAUMA, AND GRIEF

# DAY 30. SOOTHING RAGE: TAMING THE ANGRY DRAGONS

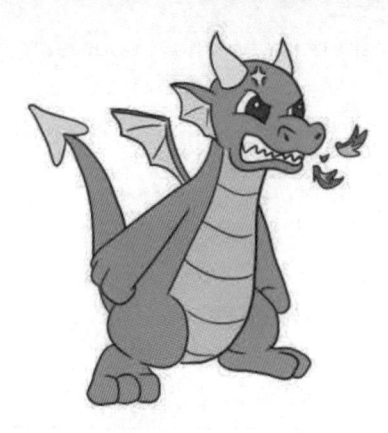

You were hurt, shamed, bullied, abused, or disappointed; or perceived you were hurt, shamed, or disappointed by others.

| COMMON WHEN... | TRIGGERS | REACTIONS | STRATEGIES | AFFIRMATIONS |
|---|---|---|---|---|
| Others modeled angry behavior for you. | Anything that reminds you of the hurtful, shaming, bullying, or abusive behavior of the past<br><br>Reminders of past disappointments<br><br>When others overwhelm you with words<br><br>When others want you to take responsibility for something | Irrational rage, frequent irritability, easily frustrated, rude, inconsiderate<br><br>Bullying, belittling, annoying, being disobedient, blaming, fighting, punishing, name-calling, stonewalling<br><br>Heart rate increases, sweating, cold hands, muscle tension, goosebumps, dizziness, confusion | Make a list of 10 things to do when you are angry to distract yourself.<br><br>Remember that anger can be good if it is directed positively and appropriately for present-day reasons. | I express my anger in ways so that others can hear.<br><br>I accept responsibility if my anger has hurt someone.<br><br>I direct my anger appropriately.<br><br>I do not use anger to scare or frighten other people.<br><br>I express my anger in words, never physical actions, unless someone I love is threatened. |

**Day 30 Exercise: Distract yourself.**

*Place a checkmark next to the following ways you will distract yourself when you get angry.*

- ☐ Consciously focus on your goals for the situation.
- ☐ Be aware of your own danger signs before your anger is about to blow. When you feel these symptoms, take 10 deep breaths (3 seconds in; hold for 1 second; 6 seconds out; hold for 1 second), which takes less than 2 minutes. You will express your feelings in a more effective way afterward—guaranteed!
- ☐ Put your hands in warm water.
- ☐ Listen to soothing music.
- ☐ Take a walk or exercise to release some of the excessive energy.
- ☐ Take a shower or bath to wash off the negative feelings.
- ☐ Journal your negative thoughts to get them out of your head and evaluate them (see Day 7 and Day 36).
- ☐ Keep a lavender sachet and inhale the aroma with five deep breaths when upset.
- ☐ Eat a healthy snack in case you are hungry because your blood sugar is low.
- ☐ Call a friend.

*Note: To calm the Angry Dragons, be sure to find out if you've had a head injury. Healing any damage to your brain can help you soothe the Angry Dragons.*

# DAY 31. BEHAVIOR IS MORE COMPLICATED THAN YOU THINK: TAMING THE JUDGMENTAL DRAGONS

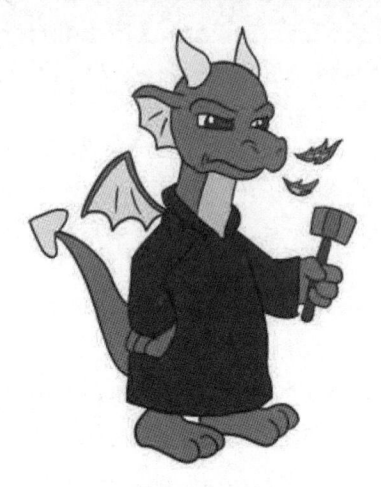

Grew up in an environment where you were hurt or perceived life was unfair.

| COMMON WHEN... | TRIGGERS | REACTIONS | STRATEGIES | AFFIRMATIONS |
|---|---|---|---|---|
| People played favorites.<br><br>People were inconsistent in how they applied rules.<br><br>You were left out of activities.<br><br>You were left out of important decisions. | Whenever you feel injustice to yourself or others<br><br>When you see others doing something you think is wrong | Condescending and critical<br><br>Moralizing and correcting people<br><br>Telling others what they should and shouldn't think or do | Ask questions when you feel judgmental.<br><br>REACH (Day 40) for forgiveness<br><br>Be curious, not furious.<br><br>Ask yourself if you are actually feeling insecure.<br><br>Judge behaviors, not people.<br><br>Get out of your bubble. | I trade judgment for understanding.<br><br>I release judgment so I can feel free.<br><br>I treat people in pain with compassion, not more pain.<br><br>I am a role model for what I want to see in the world.<br><br>I foster peace in this situation so there will be more peace in the world. |

***Day 31 Exercise: Ask questions and be curious, not furious.***

If I'm feeling judgmental today, I will ask questions:
- ☐ Is the problem from the present, or am I trying to right a wrong from the past?
- ☐ Do I have all the facts?
- ☐ Am I making assumptions about others?

Be curious, not furious.
- ☐ Help someone you would normally judge.
- ☐ See them for who they were and how they grew up.
- ☐ See if the help is for them, but the healing is for you.

# DAY 32. IF IT IS MEANINGFUL I DO IT: TAMING THE DEATH DRAGONS

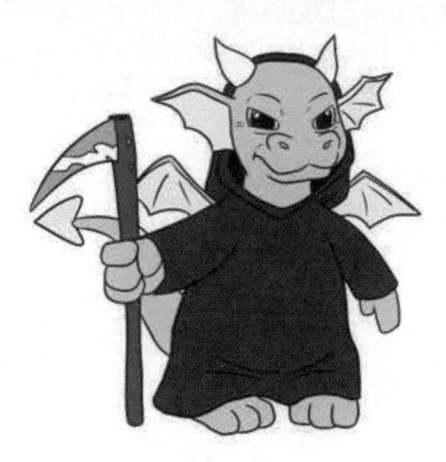

This dragon is always with us and often rears its head during midlife or earlier if you have to confront death.

| COMMON WHEN... | TRIGGERS | REACTIONS | STRATEGIES | AFFIRMATIONS |
|---|---|---|---|---|
| Your spouse leaves you for a younger person.<br><br>You have a health scare.<br><br>You start having trouble in the bedroom.<br><br>Your parents or a friend dies.<br><br>Aging or losing your youth.<br><br>Feeling life isn't meaningful.<br><br>Fearing others won't survive without you. | Pandemics, illness, funerals, near-miss incidents, losing friends or loved ones<br><br>Looking in the mirror and seeing wrinkles or other signs of aging | Fear of aging or dying preoccupies your thoughts<br><br>A pervading sense of doom or panic attacks<br><br>Physical illness (hypertension, heart disease, gastrointestinal issues)<br><br>Risky behaviors that are potentially deadly | Create a list of what you want to accomplish during your life.<br><br>Focus on issues that have eternal value.<br><br>List good things about dying.<br><br>Get your brain and body right. | I will live a life that matters.<br><br>I will live life fully and fearlessly.<br><br>I will be present today in all I do.<br><br>Death teaches me that if something is meaningful I do it, but if it is not meaningful I do not do it.<br><br>Death is just the next stage of eternal life. |

**Day 32 Exercise: Know what you want to accomplish and list good things about dying.**

The Death Dragons are always with us and often rear their head during midlife or earlier if you have to confront death. One of the best ways to tame the Death Dragons is to optimize the health of your brain and body. Another helpful strategy is to create a list of what you want to accomplish during your life. Be sure to make it meaningful and choose activities that support your values and relationships.

*In the chart below write down what you want to accomplish in life and how they fit into your values.*

### WHAT I WANT TO ACCOMPLISH IN MY LIFE

| I WANT TO... | HOW DOES THIS SUPPORT MY VALUES AND RELATIONSHIPS |
|---|---|
| Be a Brain Warrior role model for my daughter and nieces | Will enhance my own brain health and strengthen our relationships |
| Do more public speaking and write more books | Helps spread the word about brain health |
| Grow our Brain Warrior tribe | Will help our society and future generations |

| I WANT TO... | HOW DOES THIS SUPPORT MY VALUES AND RELATIONSHIPS |
|---|---|
|  |  |
|  |  |
|  |  |
|  |  |
|  |  |

*In the chart below, list the good things about dying.*

| GOOD THINGS ABOUT DYING |
|---|
|  |
|  |
|  |
|  |
|  |

Example: Here are 5 things on Dr. Amen's list.

| DR. AMEN'S GOOD THINGS ABOUT DYING |
|---|
| My faith leads me to believe in eternal life and I may get to see my father and grandfather again. |
| No more clogged toilets or running out of toilet paper. |
| No more root canals or dentists poking around my mouth with drills and other sharp metal objects. |
| Benjamin Franklin said, "In this world nothing can be certain, except death and taxes." So after death, no more worries! |
| When I'm cremated, I'll have a smoking hot body. |

# DAY 33. FINDING JOY AGAIN: TAMING THE GRIEF AND LOSS DRAGONS

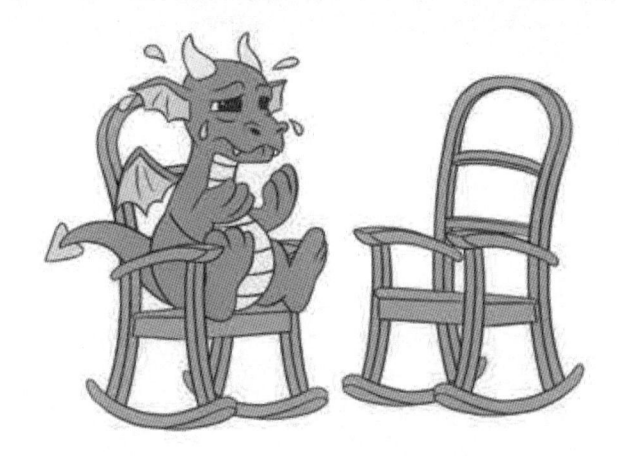

Grief and Loss Dragons are easy to find because they are everywhere, especially after the coronavirus pandemic.

| COMMON WHEN... | TRIGGERS | REACTIONS | STRATEGIES | AFFIRMATIONS |
|---|---|---|---|---|
| You lose someone important (death, divorce, a partner with dementia, empty nest syndrome).<br><br>You lose something important (health—mastectomy, a job, a beloved pet).<br><br>You lose an attachment to ideas or what could have been. | Anything that reminds you of the loss<br><br>Seeing something that brings up memories<br><br>Hearing something, such as a song<br><br>A routine that takes you back | Shock, sadness, denial, despair, anger, guilt, loneliness, helplessness, yearning<br><br>Anxiety<br><br>Sleeplessness<br><br>Memory loss<br><br>Physical sensations (trouble breathing) | Start the healing process ASAP.<br><br>Turn 5 stages of grief upside down.<br><br>Brain healthy routine: fix sleep first, supplements, social support, belly breathing.<br><br>Be on the alert for an ANT invasion.<br><br>Write the story of what happened.<br><br>Remember the positive, make peace with the rest. | I feel my feelings and cry when needed.<br><br>I choose to heal and move forward.<br><br>I hold on to love, let go of grief.<br><br>The strong person seeks help when in need, not the weak one.<br><br>Even though I'll never be the same, it is okay to be someone new. |

SIX WEEKS TO OVERCOME ANXIETY, DEPRESSION, TRAUMA, AND GRIEF

*Day 33 Exercise: Remember the positive, make peace with the rest.*

Grief and Loss Dragons are easy to find because they are everywhere, especially since the coronavirus pandemic hit. Too often, when we lose someone, we tend to remember the good times and completely ignore the bad ones. In reality, most people have conflicting feelings about the important people in their lives. Remembering an unbalanced situation prolongs grief.

*Think of someone (or something) you have lost and write down the positives that trigger good memories and the things you need to make peace with. You don't need to have the same number of memories in each column. Depending on your relationship, you may have more positives or more things to make peace with.*

*Example: Here are a few ways Tana remembered her conflicted feelings about her late father.*

| POSITIVES | MAKE PEACE WITH |
|---|---|
| At the end of his life, he made an effort to get healthier. | He abandoned me when I was a young child. |
| He overcame depression by adopting a healthier lifestyle. | He was a drug addict. |
| He had a repentant attitude about his shortcomings. | He was unpredictable. |

| POSITIVES | MAKE PEACE WITH |
|---|---|
|  |  |
|  |  |
|  |  |
|  |  |

# DAY 34. FINDING HOPE: TAMING HOPELESS AND HELPLESS DRAGONS

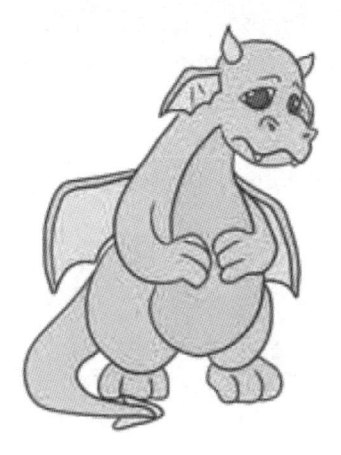

These dragons feed depression, withdrawal, and even suicidal thoughts

| COMMON WHEN... | TRIGGERS | REACTIONS | STRATEGIES | AFFIRMATIONS |
|---|---|---|---|---|
| You have tried to change your circumstances in the past, but it never worked out. You don't believe you can change your situation. You have a low sense of self-efficacy. | Situations that remind you of feeling overwhelmed. Situations that remind you of feeling powerless | Depression, negative mind-set, high negativity bias. Social withdrawal. Feelings of hopelessness, helplessness, powerlessness. Blaming yourself and others. Lack of self-efficacy | Create a positivity bias. Train your brain in gratitude. Write down your accomplishments and strengths. Get your brain healthy. Kill the ANTs. | I am worth it. I can ask for help when I need it. I have hope for the future. Today is going to be a great day. What went well today? |

SIX WEEKS TO OVERCOME ANXIETY, DEPRESSION, TRAUMA, AND GRIEF

*Day 34 Exercise: Create a positivity bias and train your brain in gratitude.*

**1. Create a positivity bias.**

Purposefully start each day on a positive note. As soon as you awaken or your feet hit the floor in the morning, start the day by saying, "Today is going to be a great day" out loud. Since your mind is prone to negativity, unless you train and discipline it, it will find stress in the upcoming day. When you direct your thoughts to "Today is going to be a great day" your unconscious brain will help you uncover the reasons why it will be so.

Tomorrow morning (and every morning after that) when you wake up, say:

## "Today is going to be a great day."

Likewise, at the end of the day, write down or meditate on "What went well today?" Doing this will set up your dreams to be more positive, giving you a better night's sleep.

Tonight (and every night after that) when you go to bed, ask:

## "What went well today?"

**2. Train your brain in gratitude.**

Being grateful for what you have can be so helpful in taming the Hopeless and Helpless Dragons. Take gratitude to the next level by adding an accountability element. This helps keep you in a more grateful mind-set.

Choose a "gratitude buddy" and commit to texting (or emailing or any other form of communication) each other at least once daily with your list of what you're grateful for.

My gratitude buddy: _____

# DAY 35. IT'S NOT ALL ABOUT ME, BUT ABOUT GENERATIONS OF ME: TAMING THE ANCESTRAL DRAGONS

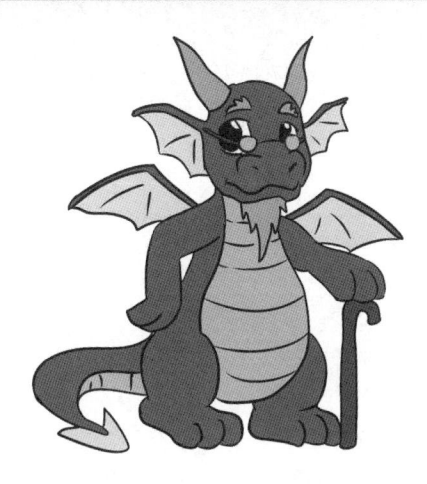

These are your parents' or grandparents' issues passed down to you through their genes, behaviors, or cultural expectations. Their anxieties, fears, prejudices, preconceived notions, political affiliations, and more become yours.

| COMMON WHEN... | TRIGGERS | REACTIONS | STRATEGIES | AFFIRMATIONS |
|---|---|---|---|---|
| You're a child or grandchild of trauma survivors (the Holocaust, 9/11, genocide, massacres, slavery, abandonment, war).<br><br>A loved one died by suicide.<br><br>You lived in a war zone.<br><br>You experienced the early death of a child/parent/sibling.<br><br>A parent had PTSD. | Being the age of a parent or grandparent when they had their trauma<br><br>Cultural expectations (often unknown)<br><br>Thinking what you should do to make your family proud or accepting of you | Reluctant compliance<br><br>Rebellion<br><br>Feeling guilty<br><br>Feeling like you are a disappointment<br><br>Anxiety for little to no reason<br><br>Unexplainable fears | Know your family history in detail.<br><br>Work to separate ancestors' issues from your own.<br><br>Reduce exposure to triggers.<br><br>Design a new future.<br><br>Try Somatic Experiencing. | I appreciate and honor my ancestors.<br><br>Sometimes my anxiety may not be from my lifetime but another lifetime.<br><br>I work to live in the present and the future. |

**Day 35 Exercise: *Know your family history.***

Are your issues from another generation? To discover your Ancestral Dragons, learn as much as possible about your family history. Talk to your parents, grandparents, and whoever is the family historian about your ancestors' biggest traumas and challenges. It can help you understand some of your automatic reactions that seemed puzzling to you before. Work to separate your ancestors' issues from your own issues, so that you can live in the present rather than the past. This may require professional help.

In the chart below, jot down some of the best and worst moments of your ancestors' lives and the dragons they may have fueled to help you recognize your Ancestral Dragons. We've included charts for your mother, father, and grandparents, as well as several additional blank charts that you can use for great grandparents, stepparents, or other ancestors (just fill in the relationship in the space provided).

*Example: Here are some of the most memorable moments from one of Tana's ancestors, her maternal grandmother Abla, whom she writes about in her book* The Relentless Courage of a Scared Child.

### Grandmother (mother's side)

| Worst | Best | Dragons |
|---|---|---|
| 1. Grew up in war-torn Syria during WWI & experienced starvation | She survived | Wounded |
| 2. Had to run into the mountains to hide from armed Turkish warriors | Didn't get captured | Death |
| 3. Got lost in the woods & was hungry, cold, & alone | She was found | Abandoned |

# MY ANCESTORS

## Mother

| Worst | Best | Dragons |
|---|---|---|
| 1. _____ | _____ | _____ |
| 2. _____ | _____ | _____ |
| 3. _____ | _____ | _____ |

## Father

| Worst | Best | Dragons |
|---|---|---|
| 1. _____ | _____ | _____ |
| 2. _____ | _____ | _____ |
| 3. _____ | _____ | _____ |

## Grandmother (mother's side)

| Worst | Best | Dragons |
|---|---|---|
| 1. _____ | _____ | _____ |
| 2. _____ | _____ | _____ |
| 3. _____ | _____ | _____ |

## Grandfather (mother's side)

| Worst | Best | Dragons |
|---|---|---|
| 1. _____ | _____ | _____ |
| 2. _____ | _____ | _____ |
| 3. _____ | _____ | _____ |

## Grandmother (father's side)

| Worst | Best | Dragons |
|---|---|---|
| 1. _____ | _____ | _____ |
| 2. _____ | _____ | _____ |
| 3. _____ | _____ | _____ |

## Grandfather (father's side)

| Worst | Best | Dragons |
|---|---|---|
| 1. _____ | _____ | _____ |
| 2. _____ | _____ | _____ |
| 3. _____ | _____ | _____ |

## MY ANCESTORS

**Ancestor** _____

| **Worst** | **Best** | **Dragons** |
|---|---|---|
| 1. _____ | _____ | _____ |
| 2. _____ | _____ | _____ |
| 3. _____ | _____ | _____ |

**Ancestor** _____

| **Worst** | **Best** | **Dragons** |
|---|---|---|
| 1. _____ | _____ | _____ |
| 2. _____ | _____ | _____ |
| 3. _____ | _____ | _____ |

**Ancestor** _____

| **Worst** | **Best** | **Dragons** |
|---|---|---|
| 1. _____ | _____ | _____ |
| 2. _____ | _____ | _____ |
| 3. _____ | _____ | _____ |

**Ancestor** _____

| **Worst** | **Best** | **Dragons** |
|---|---|---|
| 1. _____ | _____ | _____ |
| 2. _____ | _____ | _____ |
| 3. _____ | _____ | _____ |

**Ancestor** _____

| **Worst** | **Best** | **Dragons** |
|---|---|---|
| 1. _____ | _____ | _____ |
| 2. _____ | _____ | _____ |
| 3. _____ | _____ | _____ |

**Ancestor** _____

| **Worst** | **Best** | **Dragons** |
|---|---|---|
| 1. _____ | _____ | _____ |
| 2. _____ | _____ | _____ |
| 3. _____ | _____ | _____ |

# DEVELOP RELENTLESS COURAGE

When you take responsibility for your life and use the tools and strategies in this program to prevent or eliminate your BRIGHT MINDS risk factors and to tame your Dragons from the Past, it can help you overcome your emotional issues.

For many people, it's these final 7 days of this program that are the most life-changing. They show you how to develop the relentless courage you need to transform your life to something you never dreamed was possible.

# Week 6

# DAY 36. MASTER ANT KILLING: CHALLENGE YOUR 100 WORST THOUGHTS

On Day 7, you learned how your brain is always listening to the ANTs (Automatic Negative Thoughts) that fuel your dragons and steal your happiness. Today, you're going to discover how to master ANT killing.

***Day 36 Exercise: Challenge 100 of your worst thoughts to change your life.***

*Use the "Kill the ANTs" booklet to write down and challenge 100 of your worst thoughts using the 5 questions you learned on Day 7. When you challenge these thoughts, you can tame your dragons and create more positivity in your life. Get started by practicing how to kill the ANTs here. Write down a negative thought and ask yourself the 5 questions.*

**ANT:** _____

**ANT Type (s):** _____

### 5 Questions

*Is it true?* ____

*Is it absolutely true with 100% certainty?* ____

*How do I feel when I believe this thought?*

_____

_____

*How would I feel if I couldn't have this thought?*

_____

_____

*Turn the thought around to its exact opposite, and then ask if the opposite of the thought is true or even truer than the original thought.*

_____

_____

*Use this turnaround as a meditation.*

_____

# DAY 37. WRITE YOUR STORY TO TAME TRAUMA

When you've experienced trauma, loss, or tough situations, especially as a child, it can cast a shadow on the rest of your life. But you don't have to stay stuck in the painful past. Writing your story is a strategy that's often used in therapy that can be very helpful in overcoming trauma. Putting the story of your life down on paper is so powerful it can literally change your life. Looking at your life in a balanced way that includes not only the challenges and traumas you have experienced but also the happy moments can be beneficial in coping with past hurts and in taming dragons.

This unique therapy, which is called Narrative Exposure Therapy (NET), encourages you to relive the emotions of the events while remaining rooted in the present. Multiple studies show this psychotherapy for trauma and can be effective. When Tana wrote her book *The Relentless Courage of a Scared Child*, she found it to be very healing. Here's how you can do it.

**Day 37 Exercise: Write the story of your life.**

**1. Get it out of your head.** Think back to each year of your life (and even to before you were born) and jot down the best moments and the worst moments and the dragons they may have fueled. For ages when you were too young to remember, ask a family member if they recall your highs and lows at that age. And find out about your mother's experiences during pregnancy that might have impacted you.

**2. Gain perspective.** . Highlight the best of the best events and the worst of the worst events that have had the biggest impact on your life and have fueled your dragons.

**3. Ask for clarification.** The way you remember traumatic events may be true, but it may not be the whole story. Talking to others in your family about the trauma can help complete the picture opening. When you interview others, don't interrupt them and try not to be judgmental. Let them tell the story from their perspective.

**4. Choose how your story ends.** When you write your story, you get to be the author of your life.

**Helpful hint:** Consider using a 3-ring binder for your story so you can add pages or information as you learn more details. You'll likely find that as you talk to others, it triggers additional memories you may have forgotten.

*Example: Here are a few excerpts from the story of Tana's life as told in* The Relentless Courage of a Scared Child.

| <u>Age</u> | <u>Worst</u> | <u>Best</u> | <u>Dragons</u> |
|---|---|---|---|
| 2 | Left at home alone | Mom came home to find me | Abandoned |
| 3 | Sinking under the water in a pool | My dog Oso pulling me out | Wounded |
| 4 | Uncles doing drugs in my home | My Uncle Ray-crazy but kind | Abandoned |

# THE STORY OF MY LIFE

| Age | Worst | Best | Dragons |
|---|---|---|---|
| Pre-Birth | _____ | _____ | _____ |
| Baby | _____ | _____ | _____ |
| 1. | _____ | _____ | _____ |
| 2. | _____ | _____ | _____ |
| 3. | _____ | _____ | _____ |
| 4. | _____ | _____ | _____ |
| 5. | _____ | _____ | _____ |
| 6. | _____ | _____ | _____ |
| 7. | _____ | _____ | _____ |
| 8. | _____ | _____ | _____ |
| 9. | _____ | _____ | _____ |
| 10. | _____ | _____ | _____ |
| 11. | _____ | _____ | _____ |
| 12. | _____ | _____ | _____ |
| 13. | _____ | _____ | _____ |
| 14. | _____ | _____ | _____ |
| 15. | _____ | _____ | _____ |
| 16. | _____ | _____ | _____ |
| 17. | _____ | _____ | _____ |
| 18. | _____ | _____ | _____ |
| 19. | _____ | _____ | _____ |
| 20. | _____ | _____ | _____ |
| 21. | _____ | _____ | _____ |
| 22. | _____ | _____ | _____ |
| 23. | _____ | _____ | _____ |
| 24. | _____ | _____ | _____ |
| 25. | _____ | _____ | _____ |
| 26. | _____ | _____ | _____ |
| 27. | _____ | _____ | _____ |
| 28. | _____ | _____ | _____ |
| 29. | _____ | _____ | _____ |
| 30. | _____ | _____ | _____ |
| 31. | _____ | _____ | _____ |
| 32. | _____ | _____ | _____ |
| 33. | _____ | _____ | _____ |
| 34. | _____ | _____ | _____ |
| 35. | _____ | _____ | _____ |
| 36. | _____ | _____ | _____ |

37.
38.
39.
40.
41.
42.
43.
44.
45.
46.
47.
48.
49.
50.
51.
52.
53.
54.
55.
56.
57.
58.
59.
60.
61.
62.
63.
64.
65.
66.
67.
68.
69.
70.
71.
72.
73.
74.
75.
76.
77.

78.
79.
80.
81.
82.
83.
84.
85.
86.
87.
88.
89.
90.
91.
92.
93.
94.
95.
96.
97.
98.
99.
100.

# DAY 38. OVERCOME TRAUMA BY FINDING YOUR PURPOSE

The key to overcoming grief and trauma is finding your purpose. As Tana writes in her book *The Relentless Courage of a Scared Child*, finding her purpose helped her go from being a scared child to becoming a leader in our Brain Warrior movement.

**Day 38 Exercise: Answer the following 6 questions to find your purpose.**

**HOW TO FIND YOUR PURPOSE**

*1. Look inward.* What do you love to do? (Examples include writing, cooking, design, creating, speaking, teaching, etc. What do you feel qualified to teach others?)

*2. Look outward.* Who do you do it for? How does your work connect you to others?

*3. Look back.* Are there hurts from your past that you can turn into help for others? (Turn pain into purpose.)

*4. Look beyond yourself.* What do others want or need from you?

*5. Look for transformation.* How do they change as a result of what you do?

*6. Look to the end.* Psychiatrist Elizabeth Kubler-Ross, in her book *On Death and Dying*, said, "It is the denial of death that is partially responsible for people living empty, purposeless lives; for when you live as if you'll live forever, it becomes too easy to postpone the things you know that you must do." Ask yourself, does this worry, problem, moment have eternal value? When you die, how do you want to be remembered?

Example: When I answer these 6 questions, it looks like this:

> 1. I love working with patients, looking at brains, writing, teaching, inspiring, and creating a revolution!
>
> 2. I do it for myself, for my family, and for those who come to our clinics, read our books,

> watch our shows, buy our products, and are a part of our community.
>
> 3. My first wife tried to kill herself, which led me on a healing journey for those with mental health/brain health challenges.
>
> 4. The people we touch want to suffer less, feel better, be sharper, and have greater control over their lives.
>
> 5. People have better brains and better lives. They suffer less, become happier and healthier, and pass it on to others.
>
> 6. I want to be remembered as a husband, best friend, father, and grandfather, teacher, someone who worked to change psychiatry by adding brain imaging tools and natural ways to heal the brain, and as a leader of the brain health revolution that helped millions feel better, have brighter minds, and better lives.

Notice that only 2 of the 6 questions are about you; 4 are about others. A wise Chinese saying is: "If you want happiness for an hour, take a nap. If you want happiness for a day, go fishing. If you want happiness for a year, inherit a fortune. If you want happiness for a lifetime, help somebody." Happiness is found in helping others.

When someone asks you, "What do you do?" answer by telling them the answer to question #5.

Example: When I answer this question, I say:

I help people have better brains and better lives so they suffer less, become happier and healthier, and pass it on to others.

# DAY 39. IT'S EASY TO CALL PEOPLE BAD, IT'S HARDER TO ASK WHY

So many of us look at others who have hurt us in the past and label them as "bad." (See Day 7 for more on Labeling ANTs.) It's much harder to ask why they behave the way they do. Everybody is dealing with issues that may contribute to bad behavior. To gain a better understanding, you need to look at the lives of others in the 4 Circles (see Day 1).

*Day 39 Exercise: Think of someone you view as "bad" and view their life in 4 Circles. Circle the issues they have experienced. Chances are you'll see them in a new light and will have greater understanding of their situation.*

**BIOLOGY**
How many of the
BRIGHT MINDS
risk factors do they have?
(see Days 12-22)

**PSYCHOLOGY**
Have they experienced:
Mental health issues
Trauma
Neglect
Abuse
Grief and loss
Negativity
Lots of ANTs
Should and shaming

**SOCIAL**
Have they experienced:
Toxic relationships
Loneliness or isolation
Chronic stress
Family/friends with bad habits
Excessive negative news
Excessive social media
Divorce
Loved ones with health issues

**SPIRITUAL**
Have they experienced:
Lack of purpose
Lack of meaning of their life
Little connection to the past/future
Little connection to higher power
Lack of a moral code
Lack of accountability
Amoral mentors

# DAY 40. REACH FOR FORGIVENESS

Holding on to grudges and past hurts can fuel your dragons by increasing stress hormones that negatively impact your moods and emotional well-being. Giving grace and forgiveness can be hard, but when done properly they can also be powerfully healing. Research has linked forgiveness to mental health outcomes such as reduced anxiety and depression.

When Tana wrote her book *The Relentless Courage of a Scared Child*, she found that forgiving some of the people from her past helped her live in the present.

**Day 40 Exercise: Think about someone in your life you haven't forgiven and how it has hurt you (and others).**

How did they hurt you?

_____

_____

How do you feel about them today?

_____

_____

How do you feel when you think about them today?

_____

_____

How has your lack of forgiveness impacted your relationships with others?

_____

_____

Now, turn this around with a technique created by psychologist Everett Worthington of Virginia Commonwealth University. He has studied forgiveness for years and developed a model called REACH for forgiveness. Think about that same person or incident and reframe how you think about them.

**R = Recall the hurt.** But this time recall it differently, without feeling victimized or holding a grudge. This moves you toward relating to the offense from the point of view of the offender.

_____

_____

**E = Empathize.** Replace negative emotions with positive, others-oriented emotions. This involves empathizing, putting yourself in the shoes of the person who hurt you, and imagining what they might have been feeling.

_____

_____

**A = Altruistic gift.** Give the gift of your forgiveness to the person who hurt you. Think about a time in your past when you wronged someone and that person forgave you and remember how much freer you felt. That is your gift.

_____

_____

**C = Commit to the forgiveness that you experience.** Making a public statement of your forgiveness shapes your internal reality. Cement your feelings by engaging in a ritual such as completing a forgiveness certificate, or writing a word symbolizing the offense in ink on your hand and then washing it off.

_____

_____

**H = Hold on to the forgiveness.** If/when you encounter the offender, you may feel anger and fear, and you may worry that you haven't really forgiven them. This is just your body's response as a warning to be careful, not a lack of forgiveness.

_____

_____

**Know the 7 Cs of Relationships**

Forgiving people doesn't mean you have to let them be a part of your life today. In his book *People Fuel*, Dr. John Townsend lists 7 types of people in your life:
1. Coaches (mentors)
2. Comrades (very close friends and loved ones)
3. Casuals (friends)
4. Colleagues (coworkers)
5. Care (they depend on you)
6. Chronics (they always have issues)
7. Contaminants (they desire to damage others, controlled by their Angry Dragons)

Do what you can to eliminate the Contaminant people and increase types 1–4. This is part of self-care and will bring better balance to your life.

***Day 40 Exercise: Evaluate the people in your life: List the closest people in your life and indicate which type of "C" they are.***

| PERSON | WHICH "C" ARE THEY? |
|---|---|
|  |  |
|  |  |
|  |  |
|  |  |
|  |  |

# DAY 41. FINDING YOUR VOICE: LEARNING TO BE ASSERTIVE

To overcome anxiety, depression, trauma, grief, or any other issue in your life, you need to find your voice. It's important to say what you mean. In that way, assertiveness and communication go hand in hand. Being assertive means you express your thoughts and feelings in a firm yet reasonable way, not allowing others to emotionally run over you, and not saying yes when that's not what you mean. Assertiveness never equates with becoming mean or aggressive.

Here are 5 simple rules to help you assert yourself in a healthy manner.

**HOW TO FIND YOUR PURPOSE**

*1. Do not give in to the anger of others just because it makes you uncomfortable.* Anxious people do this a lot. They are so anxious that they agree in order to avoid the tension. Unfortunately, this teaches the other person to bully you to get their way. We teach others how to treat us by what we allow in our lives. Being assertive doesn't mean you have to be angry back, but don't agree simply because you're feeling anxious. When you're feeling anxious about another person's anger, it's a good time to do the diaphragmatic breathing techniques you learned on Day 9. As you breathe deeply, really think about what your opinion is and state it clearly without much emotion.

*2. Say what you mean and stick up for what you believe is right.* People will respect you more. People like others more who are real and who say exactly what's on their minds.

*3. Maintain self-control.* Being angry, mean, or aggressive is not being assertive. You can be assertive in a calm and clear way.

*4. Be firm and kind, if possible.* But above all be firm in your stance. We teach other people how to treat us. When we give in to their temper tantrums, we actually teach them the way to control us. When we assert ourselves in a firm yet kind way, others have more respect for us and they treat us accordingly. If you've allowed others to emotionally run over you for a long time, they're going to be resistant to change. If you stick to your guns, you will help them learn a new way of relating to you, and the relationship will improve. Ultimately, you will also respect yourself more.

*5. Be assertive only when it is necessary.* If you assert yourself all the time for unimportant issues, you'll be perceived as controlling, which invites oppositional behavior.

*Day 41 Exercise: Think about who you are and who you want to be. Write down 3 words that describe you now.*

| 3 WORDS THAT DESCRIBE ME NOW |
|---|
|  |
|  |
|  |

*Now write down 3 words that describe who you want to be.*

| 3 WORDS THAT DESCRIBE WHO I WANT TO BE |
|---|
|  |
|  |
|  |

# DAY 42. TAKE RESPONSIBILITY FOR YOUR LIFE

In Tana's book, *The Relentless Courage of a Scared Child,* she shares a story that literally changed her life. When she was in her 20s and recovering from cancer and depression, she went to a seminar taught by her uncle, a man she had feared when she was a child. Her uncle had been a heroin addict and attempted suicide, but after a lot of hard work, he eventually turned his life around. When her uncle saw Tana's self-pity, he asked her, "How much responsibility are you willing to take?"

Stunned, Tana said, "I can't take responsibility for cancer."

He replied, "I didn't ask you to take the blame. Responsibility is not blame. It's the ability to respond. Do you want 50% responsibility? Then you have a 50% chance to change the outcome. Or, do you want 100% responsibility. Otherwise someone or something other than you is in control."

Tana said she wanted 100% ability to respond ... and it was a light switch moment! It caused her to immediately start taking responsibility for her behavior and changed her life forever.

You have the same choice before you now. Do you want 50% responsibility for your life or 100%?

***Day 42 Exercise: Ask yourself how much responsibility you've been taking for your life.***
*1. In the first circle, indicate how much control of your life you've been giving away to others. What percentage is it?*

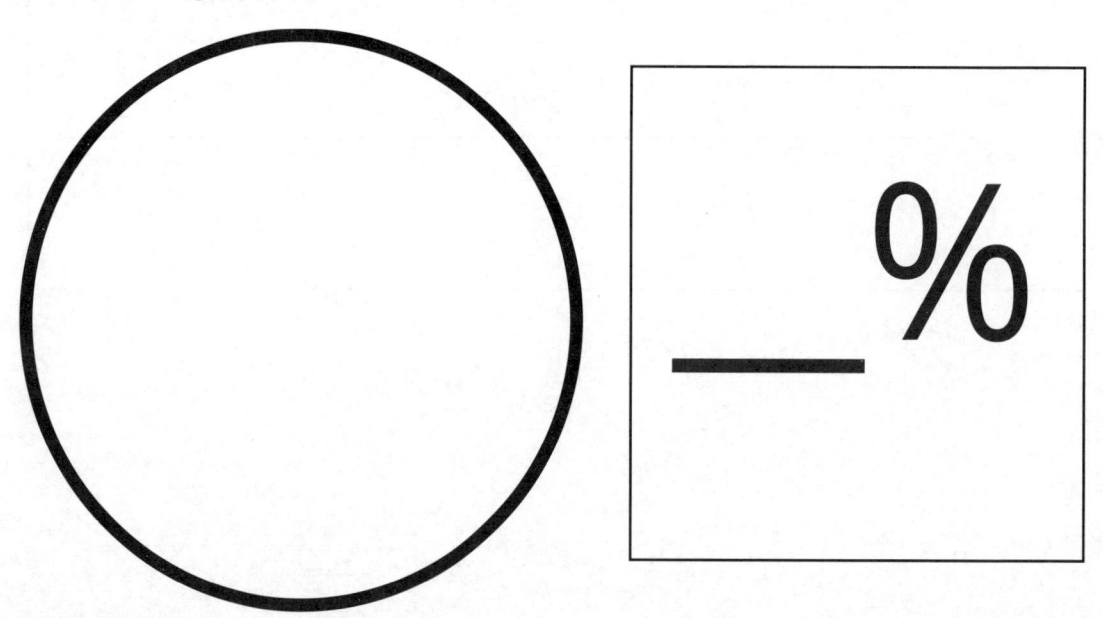

SIX WEEKS TO OVERCOME ANXIETY, DEPRESSION, TRAUMA, AND GRIEF

2. In the second circle, indicate how much responsibility you are willing to start taking. What percentage is it?

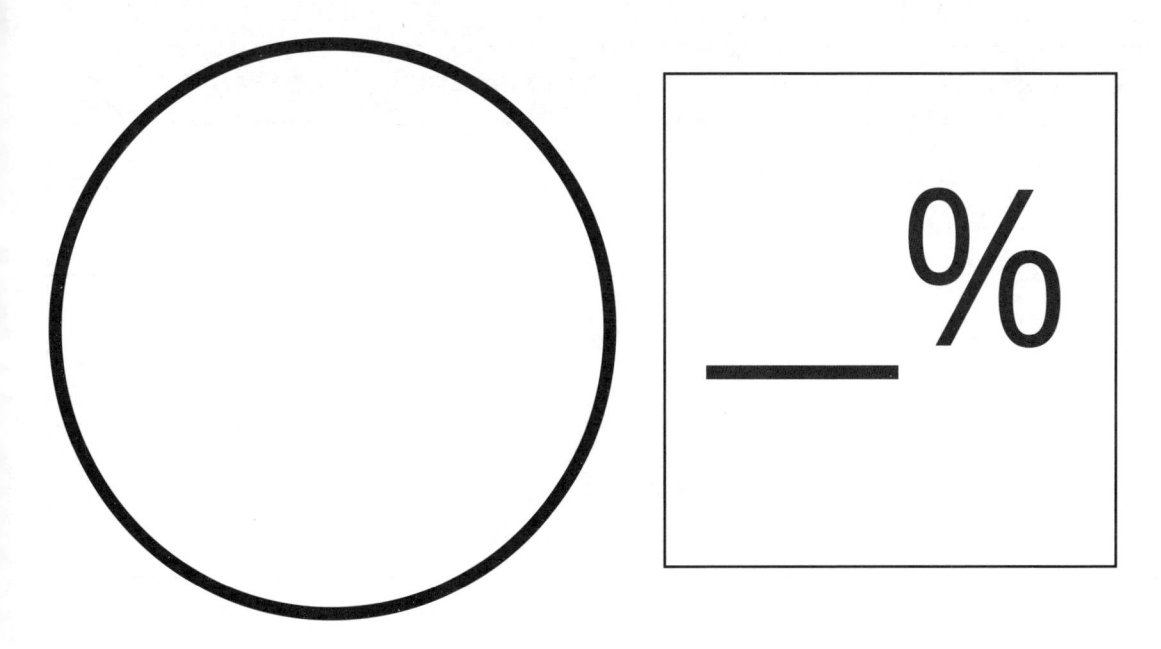

___%

Example: This is how Tana filled in the circle to indicate how much responsibility she was willing to start taking.

100%

*3. What are specific actions you will implement to take responsibility for your life? Write them down here.*

| ACTIONS I WILL IMPLEMENT TO TAKE RESPONSIBILITY FOR MY LIFE |
|---|
|  |
|  |
|  |
|  |
|  |
|  |
|  |
|  |
|  |